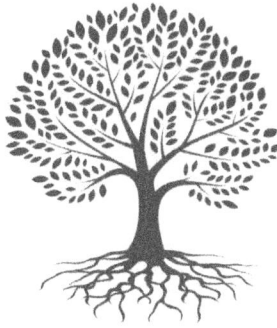

TESTIMONIALS

"Chris is one of those preciously rare people who has been able to take the tragedies in her life and use them to grow herself personally, build community for others working through their own struggles, and serve as an amazing friend and role model for those of us lucky enough to cross paths with her. She is achingly honest on bad days and brilliantly joyful on good days; always truthful, passionate, and real. Her story has lessons for all of us."

—Dr. Tina Stoeckmann
Clinical Professor, Neurologic Residency Academic Coordinator,
Department of Physical Therapy, Marquette University

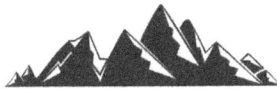

"Chris Prange-Morgan is the embodiment of true courage—not just for what she endured in her recovery from a climbing injury but for how she honestly addresses the peaks and valleys in her life in this reflective, thoughtful book. Chris brings the reader along as she thinks through the duality of many circumstances in her life. Allow Chris' experiences and knowledge to help you on your journey to better understand yourself, others, and life's challenges."

—**Janet Oberholtzer**
Author of *Because I Can*

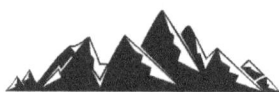

"Chris Prange-Morgan's *Broken, Brave and Bittersweet* is an unflinching examination of trauma healing as well as recovery from losses both expected and surprising. Prange-Morgan's busy life is overwhelming but doable until a rock-climbing accident changes everything she assumes about her role in the world, her body, and her relationships. Readers will find themselves quickly immersed in Prange-Morgan's wise, compassionate, and even humorous narrative as she physically and emotionally confronts her life-changing injury while reexamining what it means to parent adopted children with extraordinary needs. Prange-Morgan's background as both a social worker and community minister lends her narrative not only an authority for her topic areas but the additional vulnerability and empathy that comes with truly living what we preach. Life takes all of us down unexpected paths—*Broken, Brave and Bittersweet* is an excellent guide for the journey."

—**Joanne Nelson**
Author of *This is How We Leave*

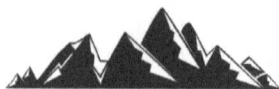

"Chris' *Broken, Brave and Bittersweet* is shockingly painful, honest, and raw. In these days of viewing parenthood and life through the lens of our social media highlight reels, Chris' story is one that validates the struggle of motherhood while embodying resiliency and dedication despite overwhelming adversity. Her growth and inner wisdom are the diamonds that emerge in these pages, and Chris' book is like a balm for anyone who has endured unrelenting struggle."

—Elizabeth Bartasius
Author of *The Elegant Out*

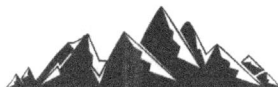

"Chris Prange-Morgan writes with honesty, wisdom, and insight about the unexpected curves that life throws at all of us. Her story is relatable to anyone who's ever had to change course suddenly, make new plans on the fly, or grow into a role they never dreamed they'd have to play."

—Larry Borowsky
Editor, *Amplitude Magazine*

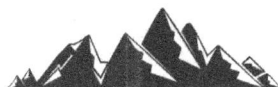

"Chris is someone who, through adversity, is able to be present with her experience, reflect on it, and grow from it. She has shown significant posttraumatic growth after her injury, a story in survival and resilience we can all learn from."

—Terri deRoon Cassini, PhD., MS.
Professor of Trauma and Acute Care Surgery,
Psychiatry and Behavioral Medicine;
Institute for Health and Equity, Medical College of Wisconsin;
Executive Director, Comprehensive Injury Center;
Director, Trauma Psychology Program, MCW;
Co-Director, Milwaukee Trauma Outcomes Project

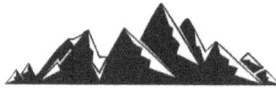

"Chris is a fellow RAD mom, survivor, and one of the most resilient people I know. Parenting a child with Reactive Attachment Disorder is not for the faint of heart. This disorder can tear a parent, and their entire family, apart. Chris has endured a series of events that most would not overcome. Chris' book is a testament to the resiliency of the human spirit and will be a 'go to' book for other struggling parents."

—Tracey Poffenroth Prato
Coach and podcast host *RAD Talk with Tracey*

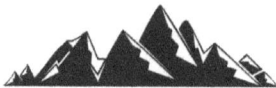

"Even though RAD is a diagnosis given to the child, it is also a family diagnosis because all are affected. The family takes the impact of the disorder: rejecting relationships at whatever cost to avoid intimacy. These actions are extreme and are traumatizing for all members of the family. We see so many families like Chris' who are desperate, lost, and parenting in overdrive. Chris' survival story is one that many parents of children with RAD can turn to as their survival guide."

—**Amy Van Tine** and **Heather Houze**
Founders and Directors of RAD Advocates

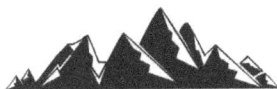

"Chris' book, *Broken, Brave and Bittersweet*, signals her willingness to fight—not in the violent sense of the word, but in the sense that she's willing to endure personal wounds so long as they eventually contribute to the benefit of others."

—**Seung Chan Lim (Slim)**
CEO, Coach, and author of *Realizing Empathy*

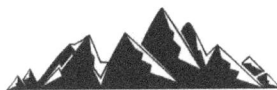

"As a Mom, I always wanted a sense of "happy, stable normal" for my family. At some point though, things don't go just as planned. Something sets you back or tosses you in a whole new direction, and we realize that our goals as parents are for something more—a family coming through the bumps of life as well-adjusted, compassionate, flexible, adaptable, even grateful people. When faced with limb loss, we experience the lows of realizing a loss, the questions of the unknown, and the challenging tasks with accepting a new normal. In time, we begin to adapt our lives and allow our children to teach us. Gratitude replaces guilt as the "me" becomes "we," and we see all that our children are capable of. These are the hidden gems in parenting children through our own limb loss. It's an often hard humble road, this one Chris and I share. But it's a deep and meaningful one, filled with opportunity, grit and profound joy."

—Kristin Hocker
Amputee mom, Maplewood Heart Foundation Director
InspirSenior Living

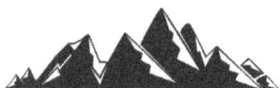

Broken,
Brave
and
Bittersweet

Broken, Brave and Bittersweet

Forging Fiercely Through Disability, Parenthood, and Other Misadventures

CHRIS PRANGE-MORGAN, MA, MSW

PYP Publish Your Purpose

For permission requests, write to the publisher, addressed "Attention: Permissions Coordinator," at the address below.

Publish Your Purpose
141 Weston Street, #155
Hartford, CT, 06141

PYP **Publish** Your Purpose

The opinions expressed by the Author are not necessarily those held by Publish Your Purpose.

Ordering Information: Quantity sales and special discounts are available on quantity purchases by corporations, associations, and others. For details, contact the publisher at hello@publishyourpurpose.com.

Edited by: Gail Marlene Schwartz, Laura Kaiser, Caroline Davis
Cover design by: Cornelia Murariu
Typeset by: Medlar Publishing Solutions Pvt Ltd., India

Printed in the United States of America.

ISBN: 979-8-88797-028-8 (hardcover)
ISBN: 979-8-88797-027-1 (paperback)
ISBN: 979-8-88797-029-5 (ebook)

Library of Congress Control Number: 2023905171

First edition, May 2023.

Publish Your Purpose is a hybrid publisher of non-fiction books. Our mission is to elevate the voices often excluded from traditional publishing. We intentionally seek out authors and storytellers with diverse backgrounds, life experiences, and unique perspectives to publish books that will make an impact in the world. Do you have a book idea you would like us to consider publishing? Please visit PublishYourPurpose.com for more information.

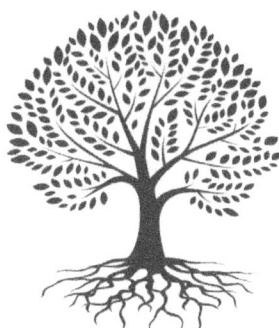

For my family.

Dad, your stubborn tenacity and athletic constitution live on.
I'll always cherish how much you've loved
and sacrificed for your family.
Thank you.

Mom, you're the reason I live by the "Golden Rule."
Even though it seems the world has forgotten
it sometimes, it's still my guide.
Thank you.

Scott, you'll always be my partner in climb.
In more ways than one, we've risen out of the ashes,
scrambled to find our feet again, and kept going.
Thank you.

Jade, I'm so proud of the beautiful young lady you've become.
Words can't express how precious you are to me.
I honor your journey and will love you forever.

Kai, you're a survivor to the core, and I'll never stop
believing in you. Do your best. Keep believing in yourself.
I'll love you always.

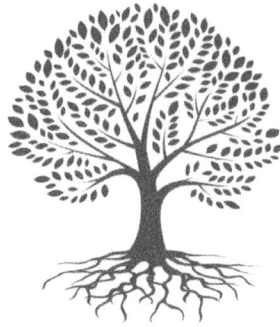

CONTENTS

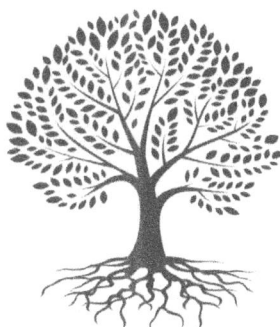

FOREWORD

I was lucky enough to meet Chris in China in 2009, when I was completing my third adoption and she was adopting her son, Kai. Right away, Chris sensed that Kai was struggling. Most adoptees exhibit delays, but Kai's delays were worse than most. Having experienced a similar situation with my first adoption, I understood what Chris was going through. I cannot describe the raw terror you feel when, in a foreign country, confronting a situation that you are completely unprepared for. Many people in this situation would choose to leave the child in China. Not Chris. Despite her fear, she straightened her shoulders and faced it head on. Chris adopted the same attitude when a climbing accident resulted in the amputation of her right foot.

With grace and determination, Chris has conquered every obstacle set before her. Hers is truly a story of hope. Now she wants to share that story with others. I have no doubt you will find hope and encouragement in Chris's story.

—**Stephanie Knipper**
Author of *The Peculiar Miracles of Antionette Martin*

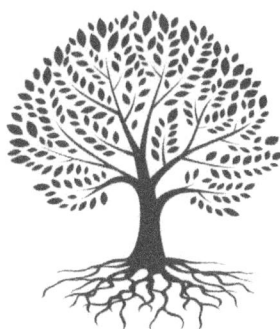

AUTHOR'S NOTE

Telling one's story and one's truth is always wrought with lots of important decisions. When sharing the intimate details of one's family life, this is even more tenuous. I spent a long time discerning whether to change the names of my family and my children before asking myself, *Why don't you just hand them your manuscript, have them read it, and ask them?*

I was humbled and surprised by the conversation that transpired with my family in their reading of these pages. I have always maintained (as you will see in these pages) that there is no shame in sharing your raw, authentic reality—because it's only through sharing these vulnerabilities that others are to liberated to do the same. No walls. No shame. Just raw humanity.

As my son wrapped up his reading of my manuscript on the last Sunday morning of winter break, I asked him to come and sit next to me on the couch in his black and red flannel pajamas, and tell me a bit about all the feels he was having. I had no idea what to expect. *Will he be angry? Sad? Resistant? Will he understand the impact of the sharing of his/my/our family story with the world?*

Kai leaned into me, took off his glasses and wiped the tears from his eyes. "I think… I'm proud," he said.

"*Proud?*" I queried, pulling him in closer, just under my arm.

"I feel like I've evolved, kinda," he declared, half-way starting to smile and laugh to keep himself from talking about the sadness.

"Stay with your feelings, Kai," I suggested. "These are important ones to feel."

He continued, "These things are hard, but they're true. Sometimes the truth is painful." I wanted to drop my coffee. He did grasp these complicated, sophisticated emotions after all.

Together, we all recalled the very hard memories within these pages. Jade agreed that our unique experiences were important enough to share without changing her name, because working through and overcoming challenges have been a huge part of her growth, as well as her life trajectory.

"These memories are part of who I am," she said. "I'm not ashamed, and I don't mind if you share them."

In the wrap up of what ended up being a very long conversation, I asked Kai to share three words that would best describe how he was feeling in that moment. He said he felt *shocked*, *amazed*, and *proud*.

"I'm shocked because I always forget about the orphanage—that I almost died," he said. "I think I feel grief too. That's hard, but I think my story can help people. I'm a real person. If you change my name, I won't feel like a real person people can relate to. I'm amazed at how far I have come. I'm proud." Tears welled up in my eyes, as I also felt pride and satisfaction with all the work we've done to get to where we are today.

Scott and I often talk about how these years of hard work have paid off, but we caution ourselves to resist the urge to think we've turned any proverbial corners. Because if we do, it seems another shrewd reality always awaits to bite us in the ass.

That very Sunday night, I awakened to some bumping around upstairs and caught my son involved in some computer shenanigans. For what felt like the thousandth time, I woke Scott from his dead-sleep to inform him of this finding.

"Yes," I said "we make progress, but *this is how it is*."

No happy endings. No huge "*hurrah!*" Just truth, hope, and persistence in working through our unique and incredibly human circumstances.

Life is humbling. This isn't a story about resolution, as much as it's a story of determination, acceptance, and resolve. It's my hope that our story (yes, of survival) will become part of another person's and/or family's survival guide.

The names of various people and professionals in this book have been changed, as well as some identifying details, situations and locations.

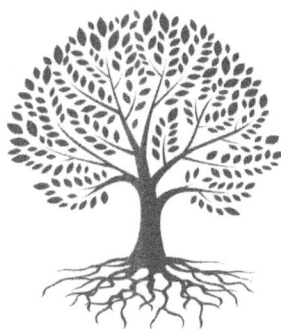

CHAPTER 1

DESIRE MEETS REALITY

As my body plunged thirty feet and crashed onto the carpeted climbing gym floor, the overwhelm caught up with me. It was too late to turn back. Shattered and broken on the floor, I knew I could not hit rewind. Feeling an odd combination of dread and somber, quiet relief, I admitted to the paramedic beside me, "You know, in an odd way, I probably needed something like this to happen."

THE PERILS OF UNBRIDLED GENEROSITY

Growing up, I loved to play hard and give freely. *The Giving Tree* by Shel Silverstein was my favorite book, and I toggled between seeing myself as both the boy *and* the tree—climbing her coarse, rugged trunk and swinging from her leafy branches. Each time I read "…and the tree was happy," I needed to pause. *Was she really?* She *had* to be, I thought. Giving and happiness were interrelated.

My Catholic upbringing underscored this reality by sharing stories of saints and martyrs. Captivated by tales of missionaries rescuing lost souls in foreign lands, I fancied myself saving the world one day. If I just kept trying, working hard, and pouring my intentions into alleviating all of human suffering, I would be happy… right?

I was the "good girl." In second grade at Holy Name School, I was proud of my modest, pink-flowered, puffy-sleeved blouse and starched white painter's pants. I was always the first one to raise my hand when Sister Dorothy called upon us to volunteer for different causes. Looking back on it now, I wonder if she was secretly trying to plant the seed of entering the convent in my developing seven-year-old brain, but at the time, sitting in the front of the class, I didn't care. Being a good girl made me feel special.

As a girl I couldn't be an altar server, so instead I helped collect and change church missals on Saturdays. When I entered sixth grade, I began volunteering at our local St. Vincent de Paul Center meal program, serving food to the poor. In seventh and eighth grade, I helped out with the Special Olympics and joined the Girl Scouts. By high school, I was working every summer as a volunteer counselor at a place called Camp Vista, a camp for children with special needs, nestled next to a small lake in the rolling hills of Wisconsin's Northern Kettle Moraine State Forest.

My college majors of education, theology, and social work continued my serial giving trend; I helped organize an International Youth Peace Camp, summer recreation department classes, and other service-learning programs. If I saw a need, I rose to meet it. Sacrifice and devotion to the greater good were as natural to me as breathing.

I carried this sunny, glass-half-full disposition into my career, my relationships, and ultimately, my mate choice. On a crisp snowy evening in January 2004, my eventual-husband Scott and I had our first date. The first thing he said to me was, "Are you sure you're okay with dating a short guy?" As he walked over from the window where he'd been standing waiting for me, he immediately noted our nearly four-inch height difference—he's not quite 5'6" and I'm 5'9". He was cute, wearing a brown plaid sweater and black scarf around his neck, smiling wryly.

"That tall, dark, and handsome thing is overrated," I responded, laughing with ease and comfort. "Hi Scott! Glad we could meet up on this frigid Monday night!"

We met on Match.com, where an algorhithm scored our compatibility tests as "*an excellent match!*" I indicated in the interests section of my profile that I enjoyed going to the dentist, cleaning baseboards, and talking to telemarketers, and listed my legs as my best physical feature. For Scott's best physical attribute, he listed his butt. Humor played a big part in our relationship, a comedy of errors from the outset.

We connected instantly; conversation flowed with ease and excitement over a glass of wine and a plate of bang-bang shrimp. I learned that we were both Enneagram sevens and ENFPs on the Myers Briggs Personality Inventory, drawn to excitement and epic life experiences, fun, and adventure (as well as the darker, flip-sided fears of being trapped, stuck, and/or in pain).

Scott shared that when he'd lived in Las Vegas years earlier, he'd picked up a passion for rock climbing in Red Rock Canyon in the afternoons to destress after a tiring day of working with at-risk kids.

"It's like I leave all my worries on the wall," he said. Being in-the-moment, in a type of "flow state," was something he loved about the sport. "When I'm climbing, I'm just focused on getting to the next hold. Not what happened earlier, not what's happening tomorrow, just sweating it out on the wall, in nature."

Our conversation morphed as we ordered a second, then third, glass of wine, jabbering on about all the adventures we'd had in our lifetimes. I learned Scott was also a "serial giver." Like me, he is the oldest child in his family and wears his "hero" hat proudly—an ascribed role we realized later had arisen from his growing up in an alcoholic family. I joked that he should have the Superman logo tattooed on his chest. He scoffed, admitting that he *had* actually considered that tattoo at one time.

We gabbed about how our jobs could get very stressful and how much we loved them, in spite of those stressors. He worked as a school psychologist and guidance counselor, and I as a social worker in the mental health field. We talked about how, as much as it sucked being the "responsible ones," it was rewarding to feel needed and valued, integral to the systems we worked within. We spoke of the relief that comes with inhabiting our bodies and being active during times of stress, how nature is healing, and how thankful we both were for being strong, gifted athletes.

"Do you do hugs?" Scott asked toward the end of the evening as we toasted one last velvety glass of Merlot.

"Of course," I chuckled, suggesting that our next date be a trip to our local climbing gym. Ideas swirled into the evening air as he walked me out to my car, gentle snowflakes drifting downward and ice crumbling underfoot. We talked about camping, climbing, and spending more quality time together—planning for more excitement and connection in the days ahead.

I felt I'd found a playmate, someone with similar inclinations and vision, but also a guy who would walk with me and grapple with all the challenges that come with living a life of such high idealism. I sensed we understood each other. Even though Scott was raised in a secular household (I jokingly called him a "heathen"), it didn't matter. Our values still clicked. I surmised that we'd continue to be compatible as we spent more and more time together, working through our penchants to chase adventure while living, giving, and loving boldly.

Like shade and sunlight, I dreamt we'd find our balance in a world that could be fun and unpredictable at the same time. While I knew our giving natures drew us to each other, I hadn't considered that the same idealism that brought us together also harbored blind spots and long-dark shadows from our pasts. I also couldn't see that the lofty naiveté we held as we professed our vows of "for better or worse" would come crashing down as the stakes got higher and higher, and we welcomed children into our lives.

We hit the ground running. At the ages of 42 and 36, Scott and I got married in Playa del Carmen, Mexico, bought a house in the 'burbs, and began the process of planning to raise a family. I miscarried once, trying to conceive the good old-fashioned way. By the time I turned 38, it was clear that continuing trying to conceive a child would be very risky. The "dream of pregnancy" wasn't something I'd ever held on to very tightly anyway. Adoption rose to the surface as what seemed most optimal for us, given our ages, resources, and life outlook. After all, there were waiting children needing homes, and our hearts were open to raising them. *Why not?* Scott and I had generosity in spades. We had years of "special needs" experience, hearts full of love, and ambition to take on whatever the universe would throw our way.

OVER THE MOON

In the summer of 2006, I began the process of looking into special needs adoptions. One photo caught my eye: that of an 18-month-old Chinese little girl, sporting a wide drooling smile, a crew cut, and an orange tank top. Her "special need" was cleft lip and palate, and her lip had already been surgically repaired. We were fortunate enough to have an amazing craniofacial surgeon at Children's Hospital, which was practically in our backyard.

I was so taken with the photo of this little toddler, who I called a "little spitfire" from the outset. Sitting in a green chair, leaning forward with her chubby little fingers grasping the wooden arm rest, I could see in her eyes that she wanted to engage with whoever was behind that camera. The bright spark of her giggly little personality reached out and tugged at my heartstrings, as if to say, "Hey Mom, I'm too playful and smart to be here, and it's cold. Please come and get me!"

Her given name was Yu Mei, meaning *beautiful Jade*, and I became obsessed with bringing her home. "Look at how she's sitting, Scott," I noted. "She's a little diva! We've got great medical insurance for her cleft. I know it's a birth defect that will take a lot of attention, but we can do this. We have to. I *know* this is our daughter!"

While Scott didn't have the same emotional attachment to the photo as I did, he slowly began to embrace the idea of moving ahead with a special needs adoption, starting the paperwork process, and bringing her home.

In January 2007, we received our approval from the China Center for Adoption Affairs. It was really happening—*wahoo!* By April, we were making plans to travel to China. Scott and I were ecstatic. We were finally going to be a family.

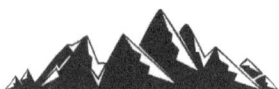

Jade came into our lives on a sunny, hot, and steamy July afternoon. Seven families congregated in the gleaming, white marbled hallway of the West Lake Hotel in Fuzhou, China, all eagerly anticipating meeting their new child.

"Look, Scott, there she is!" I noticed Jade in an instant. She was dressed in a bright pink-patterned dress with a little white t-shirt underneath, and she wore a pair of blue, red, and yellow platform Tigger sandals. Her hair was thick and freshly cut in a pageboy style, showing the nape of her neck as she turned her head from side to side. Scott grabbed my elbow and we both commented that Jade looked very healthy. She was pudgy, clean, and well-groomed. As we watched her scan the room, it was obvious that she was smart and perceptive. "She's taking it all in," Scott said.

As I had imagined, Jade was a spunky, energetic toddler with a sunny disposition and a need for constant stimulation. She gained the nickname "jumping Jade" due to her inclination to hop around like a pogo-stick and giggle. Jade loved to learn and play. In my late 30s, I had no shortage of ambition but I found I was lacking the youthful vigor I had in my younger years.

It didn't take us long to realize that sooner rather than later, with all of her exuberant and bubbling energy, she would need a sibling for companionship.

IN THE SHADOWS

You never need to apologize
for how you choose to survive.

—CLEMENTINE VON RADICS

The second time I flew to China to bring home a child was practically the opposite of the first one. It was winter 2009, another damp, cold February. In a dank, sterile government building in the hazy, polluted city of Zhengzhou, China, I was handed a wailing toddler, who was smeared in feces and wanted nothing to do with my love. I felt a strong ache in the pit of my stomach. I had waited so long from the other side of the world for this day. The precious photo of our cute, dimpled, waiting son in an oversized, puffy yellow and teal sweatshirt burned in my heart, pining for this new addition to our growing family. I'd spent so much time trying to save this child. Why was he rejecting me?

For an hour and a half, he writhed and cried without stopping, not once looking at me or my daughter. I couldn't understand. I had read all the papers about him and knew he spent most of his hours languishing in a cold orphanage crib. But I stubbornly kept thinking, *I can help him. He will attach. We will grow to love each other.* As I tried harder to connect, he continued to thrash about, resisting all eye contact, touch, or any type of warmth or connection. It became more and more apparent that this child wanted nothing to do with me. He wailed and kicked, bucking like an angry animal as I tried to wipe the tears from his sweaty, reddened face.

Jade sat beside me on the floor with an arsenal of chocolate chips, placing chip after chip into his mouth as he drooled, sobbed, kicked, and pushed away. Trying to comfort him, I tried to pull him closer to my chest with my hands gently cradling his head. He bucked back. Nothing—*nothing*—would bring him comfort. Scott walked around the room trying to obtain video footage of this momentous day as Jade and I tried to console our newest little family member to no avail. Four other waiting families were with us in this dimly lit room, which felt crowded and claustrophobic, booming with raucous emotion and chaotic overwhelm for the children and families alike. We had been handed a bundle of pent-up anguish, oozing with trauma from a two-year ordeal of despondent heartache and profound neglect.

He wiggled, pressing his feet against my chest and arching his back, shifting his center of gravity trying to escape my grip. *What is it about me?* I wondered. *Do I smell bad? Do I look funny? Has he never seen a Caucasian person before?* Sweat poured down my armpits and soaked my green turtleneck as I tried to keep him from falling out of my lap. *It will be fine,* I thought.

"All he needs is love," they told us, and I believed it. I seized the hope that I could make a difference in the life of this child who I knew had been living some kind of private hell in his hard, blue, metal-and-wood orphanage crib. I knew I could give him the nurture and warmth he'd been robbed of in his earliest days if he would just let me in.

I repeated to my husband over and over, "This is good. He's supposed to be grieving. This is all a part of the process." Scott cocked his head to the side and raised an eyebrow, shrugging his shoulders, before continuing to capture more video footage. I desperately wanted to believe that our sheer desire to love and nurture our new son would propel him into a healthy new beginning—one he surely would embrace in time.

The months prior had been laden with challenges of their own. As we spent months waiting for papers that would finalize the adoption, I happened upon a disturbing photo of our soon-to-be-son, posted by another mom in an adoption Yahoo chat group. He was around 20 months old but appeared more like an infant, scrawny-bodied, oddly larger-headed than normal, with a Band-Aid pasted to the side of his shorn head. His skin looked shriveled and pale, with his little hands and fingers dangling lifelessly. Held in the arms of a Chinese nanny, his arms and legs looked emaciated. His head rested in the crook of her arm, clearly lacking the strength to lift himself up, while his eyes stared off into the distance looking empty and resigned.

Six months earlier, I had felt elated when we finally received approval from our adoption agency saying we'd been matched with our son, whom we had seen on a "waiting child" forum. Other than a cleft lip and palate (something we were now very comfortable with), he *seemed* healthy from the low-grade photos provided. Looking at these other photos online, I felt a tugging sensation in my gut.

"Look at him," I said to my husband, pointing at the photo. "He's malnourished, Scott. He's not thriving! Oh my God, he won't make it if we don't do something. We can't let him die." My heart hurt, and my mind darted from potential solutions to contacts I could make in an attempt to get him help. I could not let him die.

I promptly called our adoption agency; they gave me the name of a woman in China whom people would hire privately to look into complicated medical situations or other areas of glaring concern for the families of children waiting for adoption. Within two weeks, she went to his orphanage and sent us his measurements, weight, and three current photos—all solidifying our concern for his wellbeing.

At 21 months old, he weighed 13.9 pounds and still could not sit unassisted. He had poor muscle tone, and his weak and lackluster demeanor led us to have grave concerns about potential underlying undisclosed health conditions, such as heart or brain abnormalities. The three photos showed our son in various positions in the arms of two caregivers, looking at the camera with his smile noticeably forced, bearing a confused expression. His skinny, lifeless arms were visibly held up by the nannies, and a recently shorn head loomed large upon a pale, skeletal, listless body.

I became more than convinced that I needed to help him somehow, even from the other side of the world. I absolutely had to get him medical help in China in order to keep him alive while we waited to bring him home. Of course, *how could I not?* Without help *he. Would. Die.* Doing nothing seemed akin to terminating a paperwork pregnancy. In seeing his obvious failing condition, I knew without a doubt that he simply could not survive if nothing was done to improve his condition. I had no idea why he looked malnourished and underdeveloped. That didn't matter. What mattered was the verification and visible evidence I now had that he needed help—fast.

I was proud of my distinct ability to sniff out human need like a bloodhound and act when the stakes were high. But I had never felt such desperation and fury. I felt caught between feelings of anger at a system I knew nothing about and resentment toward a situation I knew I did not cause but that my heart had to do something about.

I'd advocated for countless people in my job as a social worker. But I had never, ever imagined I would be using this same skillset, from the opposite side of the globe, to save a child I had seen in referral papers and pictures but had not met yet—a son who had nonetheless taken root in my heart as if connected to me by an umbilical cord.

Fortunately, Love Without Boundaries, an international charity providing necessary medical and material aid to Chinese orphanages, agreed to sponsor him and send him to a pediatric medical facility in Beijing. There, he received an evaluation, testing, and proper care and nutrition for the next three months before returning to the orphanage to prepare for his adoption.

While awaiting approval to travel for Kai's adoption, we were told some of the staff from the medical facility had serious concerns that he would actually explode from overeating. I understood that the employees were likely not medically trained and that they were caring, well-intentioned people who were simply confounded at the immense hunger response our waiting son presented with. It was their job to tend to the children and to consult with the medical staff if they had concerns about the children in their care. I had to let go of my desire to know everything (since I couldn't) and trust that his needs were finally being met in the best way they could be. He clearly had no satiation response (feeling of fullness) when being fed. Of course, babies don't explode. Still, I was afraid of what this meant for our waiting son's physical and emotional development. *What does this way of existing do to people? How would he come to us? If the extent of his malnutrition and neglect was this horrible, what would that mean for his coming into our family?* My deep worry was quickly replaced with a reflexive altruism— if anyone could help this little boy, we could. I had some understanding of the relationship between nutrition and human development, but perhaps not enough.

I dug around online and learned that "Hunger-related toxic stress can negatively affect brain development, learning, information processing, and academic achievement in children" (Schroeder, 2019). There is a definite psychological connection between the brain and the belly and the feeling of being well. And *being well* is relative. "Malnutrition in the first years of life is especially harmful, impacting physical growth, decreasing resistance to disease, limiting the size and functioning of children's brain structures, and stunting intellectual capacity" (APA, 2022).

OVER THE SEA

We decided to name our son Kai, a Polynesian name meaning "sea" or "willow tree"—both meaningful images depicting the vastness of our travels and the flexibility with which we needed to engage our entire adoption process. It was a name Scott and I arrived upon while realizing we wanted something that was easy enough to articulate, short enough to write quickly, one that would be trendy yet timeless enough to grow old with.

While unaware what particular constitution our son had or what the future would hold, I knew that there was a fair amount of the outcome I could not control, as much as I wanted to. After seeing those images of Kai online, every fiber of my being yearned to jam through our adoption paperwork to rush the process, yet this was not possible. We petitioned to the China Center for Adoptive Affairs to expedite our adoption and waited.

I am not good at waiting. Perhaps it is my stubborn German temperament. I want to exert my will upon the outcome and create solutions as quickly and painlessly as possible—so obviously, putting my trust in the process was not easy. To an extent, I knew that I needed to let go of my desire to know everything and control the outcome, because it was impossible to do so. I was on the other side of the world, for cryin' out loud.

With Kai receiving medical care, we exhaled with guarded optimism, now feeling fairly certain that at least he would *survive*. He was in a safer place with greater resources, better nutritional support, and quick access to medical services if necessary. Love Without Boundaries was also now involved with his care. This gave me a sense of comfort that I could finally let my guard down and trust that his condition would improve, at least to some degree, before his adoption. I gradually backed off and decided to trust the rest of the process.

As we readied for our travels, I created a blog to share our experiences with friends and family. We coined the name of our family's journey and adoption blog "The Adventures of the Fab Four," and I began by sharing the initial worrisome photo I had seen online. Despite these obvious glaring concerns, there was no shortage of excitement on the horizon. Scott and I envisioned an adventurous future, filled with camping, climbing, hiking, biking, and all the outdoor activities that brought us joy. With great optimism, we continued to project boundless hope and excitement into the days ahead.

Jade was excited at the prospect of having a little brother. She was curious, smart, and precocious, so she loved the idea of being mother's little helper. Not surprisingly, she was one hundred percent onboard with welcoming a younger sibling into her burgeoning world. With anticipation and excitement, Jade would ask, "Can I help decorate his room? Can I help teach him things?" Naturally, we jumped at the chance to have her share in our enthusiasm, and promptly gave her the fun responsibility of picking out toys for his new bedroom. Taking her role very seriously, she assisted in preparing for Kai's homecoming by choosing the fun primary colors of red, yellow, and blue to paint his bedroom walls and lending her handprint to the freshly painted bookcase that would stand in the corner next to his closet. She picked out several select stuffed animals to sit on his bed, and even donated her beloved rattling Elmo to the collection.

We created a little outdoor play area in the corner of our backyard with a sandbox and wooden swing set. Jade loved to mix sand, rocks, leaves, and water in a bucket to make "soup." She was beyond excited to teach Kai her recipe for this yummy concoction.

Jade had a bilateral cleft lip and palate, and we assumed then that bringing home a sibling with similar cleft issues would be easy enough for our experienced family to handle.

In the adoption world, "special needs" are usually thought of as some type of treatable medical condition. Birth defects, heart abnormalities, and other ailments are common. Some adoptees present with other developmental issues such as Down Syndrome and autism, but rarely are potential parents given information regarding the kinds of entrenched behavioral challenges that often present themselves more strongly once a child joins their permanent family. These issues are surprisingly common in children with histories of trauma, but only recently have psychologists begun to understand the impact of Adverse Childhood Experiences (ACES).

Still, all budding families hope and dream of an idealistic, unbridled future filled with richness, depth, and laughter with their children. We expect experiences of deep connection—of shared laughter, profound joy, and mutuality of relating. These are the things which I had always believed define a strong sense of family—connection, humor, togetherness.

Adoption is often as meaningful and exhilarating for the parents as it is horrifying and disturbing for the child, whose only experiences may have been ones of pain, deep despair, and loss of everything that defines their world. At the time, I hadn't ever stopped to consider this, as my own need and desire to parent remained in the forefront of my reality. Surely my ironclad will could mold our world into a picture-perfect, suburban dream.

I had no idea that a child, whose only experience has been that of extreme neglect, heartbreak, and dashed hopes, knows nothing about mutuality. They know nothing about dreams or profound joy. Their lived experience—every fiber of their being—screams overwhelming malaise and distrust. Adults are the monsters who have allowed them to weaken, wither, and wane. For some reason, perhaps due to her temperament or better orphanage conditions, Jade seemed to have an easier time trusting adults from the outset. She understood reciprocity in relationships. She was able to ask for help when she needed it, and she saw the world as a grand, exciting place. Unfortunately, this was in stark contrast to our son's experience.

When cries for hunger or discomfort go unmet, these infants and children learn one unfortunate reality: they can't rely on adults. Day after day, week after week, year after year, lying in fetid, soiled diapers, they learn to tolerate an ungodly amount of distress and must summon up the inner resolve to somehow keep going. Some children die. Others, such as Kai, languish and hang on by a thread. Lord knows how they hang on, but they do. Barely.

In 1995, Kate Blewett and Brian Woods produced a television documentary about Chinese state-run orphanages entitled *The Dying Rooms*, and watching it after we adopted Kai helped us surmise what his life may have been like. The footage was captured by bringing an hidden camera through the various dark rooms and corridors of the orphanages where the weakest and least liked children are left to die. It's the kind of documentary where the disturbing images remain in one's mind for days and weeks afterward (as they did in mine), haunting one with continued ruminations of, *this really, truly happens?* Yes, it does. We came to believe our son endured some form of horrible neglect—if not a dying room, something wretchedly similar.

SURVIVAL

I don't think it was Kai's intention to survive. In fact, the perma-scowl Kai wore in the immediate days after joining our family signified his intense disapproval of the whole ordeal. This was accompanied by an intense recoiling (and pushing away) from any form of human touch, a severe aversion to eye contact with me and others, and a strong, dangerous thrusting back of his head any time the threat of human connection intruded upon the world of isolation he'd grown accustomed to. Years later, a therapist equated Kai's early years to being psychologically underwater, surmising that Kai had grown accustomed to simply existing—of dissociating or psychologically zoning out as a form of self-protection—while he unconsciously waited to waste away. Joining a family meant entering the land of the living, which also meant engaging with the people and the world around him.

From the moment Kai was placed in my arms, I began to feel my own vital life force leaking from within my inner reserves. Brief moments of reprieve were followed by an omnipresent looming dread. From waking up to bedtime and every moment in between, our lives became a daily struggle to resist the quicksand-like inertia which exerted its gravitational pull on our energy. Parenting this child of trauma became an all-consuming, energy-draining, life-defining task.

In his initial months with us, we employed every attachment trick suggested by our adoption agency, hoping to facilitate connection. These included attempting to wear Kai in a baby sling facing me, applying sweetened vanilla lotion to his body and face, and trying to co-sleep with him in our queen-sized bed (and later, on the floor of his bedroom, next to his bed). It became pretty obvious to us from the outset that Kai wanted no part of any of these strategies. He mentally disengaged, dissociating to some far-off place in his head, becoming limp as a rag doll as I tried to wear him in the sling. Kai rejected skin-to-skin contact by forcibly pressing away and thrusting his head back. Co-sleeping was out of the question; he couldn't relax his body or mind enough to drift off to sleep. It was apparent he could not emotionally *or* physically tolerate anything resembling the intimacy of human closeness.

Everything felt forced. This experience was vastly different than when we adopted Jade, who snuggled up to me easily, looked me in the eyes, and craved constant interaction and stimulation. Despite how hard I tried, nothing seemed to work.

After dinner one evening while we were still in China, I suggested to Scott that we pull our guide, Carissa, aside to ask her all the burning questions cropping up in our heads. *Is this normal? Is it typical to see such resistance to nurture in these kids? My gut tells me something is wrong, but I can't quite put my finger on it. Do you think it's a good idea to move forward with the adoption? Are we in over our heads?*

Carissa walked with us to our hotel room, opened the door, and she placed her brown leather bag on the desk chair. Scott and I sat at the edge of the bed while she leaned back against the desk, arms clasped across her chest.

"How are you doing?" she asked. "What is it that you'd like to know from me?"

Scott looked at me and back to Carissa. "Why is Kai throwing his head back? Why is he so weak? Are you sure this is normal?"

"Oh yes," she assured. "Your son has been in an orphanage, where there are so many mouths to feed and not enough nannies. We see this all the time. Then we hear how well the children do in their loving forever homes."

"So you're telling us this is normal?" I asked. "You see this kind of thing all the time? You really think our son will be okay—that there's not something really serious going on that we're not prepared to handle?"

"Oh no," she replied. "He'll grow and learn and be a happy boy in your family. Once you get home and have a routine, and he knows you love him, you'll see him just blossom."

We wanted to believe all these things. I felt relieved when Carissa reassured us that all would be okay in time. Yet when we did return home, it became obvious that this loving family was not enough to cure Kai's entrenched behavioral issues. Once again, I researched and sought out additional resources to help him with his delays and developmental challenges while waiting for the "blossoming" we were assured would happen.

Back in Wisconsin, our new life felt more like a pediatric infirmary than a household. Even as his body grew physically more congruent with our expectations as a now fattened-up toddler, Kai was developmentally more like an eight-month-old infant with zero skills, little muscle tone, and virtually no desire to engage with the world around him. Everything—from sitting up to maintaining attention to using rudimentary language (signing, words of any type)—was way too much physical and mental effort for our little guy, so he checked out, physically, mentally, and emotionally. Lying on the carpeted floor and drooling was about all he could do. Sadly, he could not summon up the inner strength to engage, and this meddling family he was now a part of was not welcomed in his world. My heart ached. I was tired, and I wondered if I would ever again not be tired.

As a relatively new mom, I watched parents with typical kids beaming with joy as their children ran down the hill at the park and chased their siblings up the slide, while mine sat in a lump in the sandbox, swishing his hand back and forth. *Will he ever engage with life?* I wondered. *Will he ever find joy? Will I find happiness again?*

Jade's sunny disposition kept us positive. This was new and different for her, and for all she knew, her new little brother was just a bit quirky. Scott verbalized some concerns with Kai's overall developmental immaturity (which lagged much further behind what we had ever imagined), yet, like me, he exuded boundless optimism—because we were loving people with the resolve, education, and resources to do whatever it took.

I watched in frustration as everything seemed like a herculean effort for our son. Scott and I tried to inject some levity into our situation by referring to Kai as a sack of potatoes, as he was either lying on the floor, or pathetically sagging down by his torso from my hip when I attempted to hold him. Kai wouldn't grasp onto me with his arms or his legs, so he felt much heavier than he was. My back ached. I felt a constant pang of tension behind my neck and between my eyebrows from the stress of trying so hard. Day after arduous day, I would ponder which of the multitude of issues to work on.

Kai had no interest in crawling or creeping. But our therapist offered a wise suggestion: use fruit snacks as reinforcement to get him to crawl, then walk between Scott and I, and this brought some success.

Scott sat on the floor with his back against a chair on our carpeted living room floor, crinkling a plastic bag of fruit snacks. Similar to what you'd do for a pet, he picked one out and held it up. "Come on, Kai! You can do it! Come get the fruit snack!"

I perched on the bottom stair holding Kai up under the armpits of his denim overalls, about 15 feet away from the dangling treats.

"Look Kai!" I said. "Yum yum!" He giggled and pointed to his dad, showing a promising wide, dimpled smile. "Yup! Go get it buddy!" I chirped, partially wondering if I should get ready for yet another meltdown. Kai reached one pudgy hand down to the carpet, then the other, as I lowered him to the floor, grasping the straps of his overalls. Within five seconds, he crawled to the other side of the room and nabbed the fruit snack from Scott's hand.

"Yay!!!" Scott and I applauded. "You did it!"

"Moah? Moah?" Kai lisped as he signed "more," requesting additional fruit snacks. Scott threw me the bag and I emptied out another handful, knowing that we'd keep going until the bag was empty.

Progress was possible, if slow. All skills were learned on his own terms, when he was ready. The concept of making progress for its own sake was not something Kai understood; he had zero interest. He didn't experience the world as an exciting new venture, but rather, a scary, unpredictable place in which more and more was expected of him (and thus required more painful effort).

One morning, as I tried helping Kai put on his blue and yellow winter jacket, he fell into a blubbery lump on the floor. Grunting, with a scowl on his face and a look of sheer disgust, he pulled away and refused to allow me to help him. I continued trying to wrangle this unwieldy, bucking toddler in an attempt to get out the door on time, to no avail. Beads of sweat ran down the sides of my face as his refusal escalated into a full-on tantrum, thrashing and howling with each unsuccessful attempt. I just wanted to get him dressed and be on our merry way!

I ended up stomping out to the garage to warm up the car on my own, leaving my son lying on the kitchen floor in his half-donned snow gear. As the car gradually warmed, I placed my forehead on the steering wheel and cried quietly, warm tears dropping gently into my lap. I wondered how I would continue to cope with the unending onslaught of days like this stretching into the foreseeable future, and worried that I might have a nervous breakdown of my own. *This isn't how it should be,* I thought. *This is not the life I envisioned.*

Breathing slowly, I gathered myself and peered through the windshield at the screen door, where I noticed my son had plopped himself on the filthy door mat. Sighing, I opened my car door, walked into the house, and gathered him up in the lump that he was and slung him over my hip. I turned around, trudged back to the car, snapped him into his car seat, sans-winter garb, and slammed the door with a loud resounding thud.

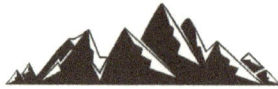

When Kai was around three, I would try to have him sit on my lap at the kitchen table. Within minutes, warm, wet urine soaked through Kai's clothing onto mine. *Shit!* I thought, *What the heck?* Initially, I thought he just couldn't control when he peed, but I began to notice that he would only urinate on me—not Dad or anyone else. It became obvious that peeing on me was a way for Kai to protest my affection. I felt a tad angry and very humiliated. *Why does he keep doing this to me?*

Tantrums and control battles could drag on for hours. This had now become our new normal. By the end of every day, I was physically and emotionally spent. So was Scott.

Each new day was more of the same. We made desperate attempts to communicate and connect. We tried using American Sign Language, signing simple words: "more" and "water" and "I'm hungry," but even these were too challenging when grunting and tantrums were his default. Jade could gain some headway by getting down on the floor with Kai and acting silly or by taking his hand saying, "Come on, Kai! Play with me!" Scott and I would break into dopey children's songs, hoping to lighten the mood, at least temporarily.

Even while still in China, we discovered that I could sneak a hearty giggle and a grin out of Kai by tickling him forcefully on his belly while he was lying on his back on the bed. His "belly laugh," as we'd call it, felt real and genuine and "normal." I wanted to feel and see and know this side of him more, to have even a faint sense of connection and levity.

The ever-doting big sister, Jade took it upon herself to teach Kai all she knew. "Here Kai, these are crayons. This one is blue, this one is orange. See? You can draw things! Maybe we can make pictures together!" Taking him by the hand, she tried to teach him words, phrases and the alphabet using colorful refrigerator magnets. "See Kai? C is for 'cat.' Can you find the yellow 'C?'" Sometimes he'd point to the correct letter, but most often not. Jade became just as frustrated as we were.

While most children want to learn to crawl, walk, and feed themselves, Kai wanted nothing to do with learning. Perhaps he felt it was too much work, especially since he had mentally checked out years ago, fully expecting to waste away in his orphanage crib. He literally hadn't planned on making it this far. Yet somehow, with her effervescent enthusiasm and dedicated confidence in her little brother, Jade was able to pique Kai's interest. She carried on in the years ahead as Kai's number one ambassador, while he chipped away at the necessary milestones to join the land of the living.

Jade's favorite show, *Sesame Street*, thankfully provided a welcome respite, even though Kai would still mentally check out, preferring to gaze at the palms of his hands or the spinning wheels of an upside-down matchbox car.

"La la la la—la la la la—Elmo's world!" Jade tried to entice Kai to sing along with her, watching Mr. Noodle's orange, bushy hair bounce.

"*I wuv Mr. Noodle!*" She'd pipe up, pointing at the TV screen.

Scott and I joked about the kids' starkly different temperaments. "She's the border-collie, and he's the sloth." Scott commented, jokingly. It was true. These characteristic images described them perfectly. I, on the other hand, felt more and more like Oscar the Grouch.

The daily routines—of teaching Kai how to express his needs, to communicate, and to *want* to engage in the world—were punctuated by occasional bright spots. I always loved Kai's dimply grin. Even though he drooled longer than any kid I've ever known (until about six months after he turned three), he would bop his head on the beat like Grand Master Flash when we keyed up Motown. Kai would sit cross-legged on the living room floor in his denim overalls and red drool-soaked turtleneck, boppin' and grooving to funk music.

"Look at Kai get his groove on," Scott would point out. My mind would occasionally drift to wondering how this life compared to his earlier moments in a cold orphanage room. *Did he even hear music back in those dark days?* This child, with his uncanny ability to catch a beat, seemed like an amazingly stark difference from that skinny boy in the photo, dangling limply in the arms of a Chinese nanny. I wondered, *Does he ever pine for the familiar sights and sounds of China? What about Jade? Does she long for her birth country?*

Daily caregiving left me with a feeling of increased isolation, underscored by a nagging sense of guilt for taking these children from everything they had known. I loved them beyond words. But something felt missing. *What's wrong?* I wondered. *Is it a biological connection? A felt sense of belonging that develops early in utero, that maybe my children will never feel?*

I felt a consistent pressure from within to portray the "normal" happy family image, always hoping no one knew I was struggling. I faked a bright, cheery smile like I had just won some coveted prize at the Parenting Games. Yet one look in the mirror, and I could clearly see the life drained from my face. Tired, dark circles formed under my eyes and a crease settled between my brows. Much of life's levity was gone, replaced with preoccupation, dread, and worry. It didn't take long for this falsely cheery pretense to become tiresome and for my energy to become completely depleted.

At night when the kids would finally be asleep, Scott and I would talk. "Honey, did you ever think it would be this hard?" I'd ask. "I'm always tired. I feel like I've lost myself."

"Me too," he'd fess up. "I know it's hard, but we'll get through it. We have to."

No one, other than Scott, understood how hard these days had become. Attempts to express this difficulty to others outside of our family were met with benign words of encouragement and decent-hearted explanations.

"Oh, the terrible twos are so hard."

"Boys are notoriously stubborn."

"Maybe he just needs a nap."

We encountered the advice-givers, the nay-sayers, and the normal-izers. They were all well-meaning, yet they had absolutely no effing clue what we were going through, since parenting a child with attachment challenges is in no way normal or intuitive. People assume connection between parent and child is inherent—that wasn't the case with our kiddo. He had never connected with anyone, and he fought with all his might to keep it that way, keeping me and everyone else far away from the protection of his isolated inner world.

No training or education had readied us for the intense feelings of aloneness we would continue to face as the family of an attach-ment-challenged, traumatized child. I had a bachelor's degree in edu-cation and two master's degrees, including one in social work, with over ten years of experience working in the mental health field. Scott had a master's degree in school psychology and almost 20 years of experience working in education. We were not inexperienced or undereducated in the topics of human development or psychology, yet we were totally caught off guard with the intensity of Kai's trauma. This was in no way typical. We had undergone the usual adoptive parenting classes and read books about toddler adoption, attachment, and intentional parenting. We had talked with dozens of adoptive parents about their experiences. While helpful, none of the training or information we had encountered had adequately prepared us for the emotional excavation and extremely gut-wrenching overhaul we would have to surmount as a family while coming to terms with the fallout of such deep orphanage neglect.

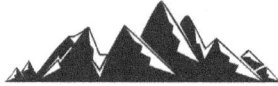

Trauma, when experienced in infancy, has the ability to permanently re-wire the brain (Child Welfare Information Gateway, 2017). Brains of neglected and traumatized children go into survival mode, and then lock in there. Since their most tender, early moments were formed in situations of broken trust, abandonment, and neglect, each subsequent relationship is met with a perceived sense of impending danger. Adults are scary and not to be trusted, even if they are the most caring and nurturing folks on the planet. Nurturing females are even more suspect since they may abandon once again, as their birth mom did. The fact that I now assumed the Mom role simply ratcheted up Kai's fear, avoidance and desire for control.

In his book *The Body Keeps the Score*, psychologist Bessel Van der Kolk says that,

> If an organism is stuck in survival mode, its energies are focused on fighting off unseen enemies, which leaves no room for nurture, care, and love. For us humans, it means that as long as the mind is defending itself against invisible

assaults, our closest bonds are threatened, along with our ability to imagine, plan, play, learn, and pay attention to other people's needs. (2015, 76)

It took lots of head scratching, learning, and working through my own denial to finally understand this truth—that trauma fundamentally changes the brain, its perceptions, connections, and all interactions with other human beings. Since my reference point was my own experience (one in which I was wanted and raised in an intact, loving family from gestation onward), I projected my assumptions onto my own children. Most of us project our own realities onto what we see. It's totally normal. And it was totally normal for me to keep hoping and waiting for my child to warm up. To turn the corner and soften. To accept my love and affection—and for me to be let down, again and again.

Motherhood felt like a contest I was ill-equipped to enter. I endured by continuing to tread water, struggling hard to not drown, and suffocating in my feelings of exhaustion, worry, and overwhelm (of course, wearing a smile to conceal the fatigue.) We just gutted. it. out.

One afternoon during one of Kai's two-hour meltdowns, I found myself retiring to the basement with a drink in hand, blasting the angst-ridden tunes on Alanis Morrisette's *Jagged Little Pill* CD. Slowly, I began to chill. And let go.

NO CONSOLATION

One of the most challenging aspects of parenting Kai was my inability to console him. His rages seemed to come out of nowhere. Often they would be prompted by an expectation of some sort—such as being asked to verbally express what he wanted or a utilize a new skill he had acquired—which didn't jive with his preferred way of being at the time (usually, laying in a silent lump on the floor). The early weeks and months of exhausting myself in an attempt to provide comfort eventually receded into a kind of resigned acknowledgment that my efforts were futile. All I could do to let go was to take solace in the realization that I did not *cause* this and rest in the acceptance that Kai's deep, aching pain came from a dark place in his past—the shadowy years and moments of waiting without hope for someone to care.

As Kai strongly railed against snapping himself in his car seat one autumn afternoon, Scott commented that if we didn't find some way to help him emotionally, he would "probably commit suicide by the time he's twelve years old." Kai's despondency was palpable and raw, and his mood shifted from anger to sadness within the course of moments. Gradually, this improved over the years, as his overall disposition became less surly (with the help of medication). It took great effort and a village—and my almost giving up in the process.

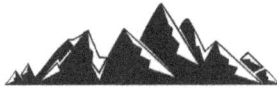

Before I got married and began raising a family, I worked for over ten years as a case manager, therapist, and social worker in Philadelphia and Milwaukee. My caseload consisted of mothers recovering from substance abuse and their children. In both cities, my clients were disproportionately people of color, poor, and often suffering multiple generations of systemic neglect in the decaying inner cities.

I knew I had seen that same hard, checked-out stare before in other kids. Similar to my son's beginnings, many children of the moms in the halfway house I'd previously worked at had been schlepped from unsafe home to unsafe home. Many of the kids had been exposed to drug use. Some had been present when their mothers engaged in sex work to earn money to support their drug dependence. Often these children were left with strangers or abandoned for long stretches of time. When these women finally came into treatment, *they* were on the road to healing, but their children had also suffered tragically along the way. Many had developed behavioral problems and mood disorders. One pair of siblings acted out sexually and needed additional treatment from specialized mental health services to keep the rest of the children in the house safe. I couldn't help but notice how similar the looks on these children faces were to my son's. There was a hardness and fear hidden behind a darkness in their eyes. Both Kai and these children knew unimaginable sorrow.

I appreciated the parenting classes these kids' moms engaged in, and I felt grateful for their hard work and tenacity in following their treatment plans during the six months the women were with us. Thankfully, these women learned skills to support and challenge one another in their parenting while also working through their own generational family traumas and the role those unresolved traumas played in fueling their addictions. By the time these ladies graduated from the treatment program, they beamed with pride at their learnings. They developed the skills to stay clean and sober while becoming better moms in the process. Of course, this took time—and a village.

I longed for a village as I raised my children. In the isolation of parenting Kai, my thoughts returned to the women and clients I had once worked with and the traumas they had endured. I couldn't help but think about the ways they had been fundamentally changed by trauma in their early lives, long before their addictions and other problems developed, and subsequently wonder how their children and grandchildren would be impacted in the years to come.

It was hard for me to truly understand the magnitude of the challenges these families had faced. My reality was so different. I had never really stopped to consider how horrifying and disturbing it can be for a child to be taken away from all they know in the most vulnerable years, whether they'd been given up for adoption at infancy or experienced instability and inconsistency in their youth. My reference point was my own lived experience, which was very different.

Still, the reality of our failing systems and the trauma those failures inflict hit me hard. I knew without a doubt that these failures lead to trauma. China is a society grappling with rapid economic changes, deep income inequality, and massive infrastructural challenges—a lot like the problems presented here in the cities. In each case, the government has priorities that exclude so many vulnerable populations. Both groups are dealing with trauma because of massive sub-optimal systems.

I came to a passive acceptance of the ubiquity of trauma. I had no idea before I brought him home that the child who had just entered our lives had so suffered greatly under a massively sub-optimal oppressive system, which had been entrenched in generations upon generations of communist policy. Prior to becoming a social worker, I had no idea that my clients' situations would be as entrenched in systemic failures—or that those kinds of systemic failures were still such a problem here in America. I learned the hard way that their lives had largely been torn apart by multigenerational poverty, decades of racial discrimination, and progressing urban decay. I ultimately came to realize that my little contribution to raising my son would be a ripple in the ocean of the world's traumas. Healing myself and our family was the best I could do.

Similar to the women in treatment for substance abuse, I would have had to acknowledge my overwhelm in order to move past it, but my stubbornness and pride kept me from doing so. I could have utilized the serenity prayer popular in AA and NA, which offers up one's will to a higher power and asks for the grace to accept the things we cannot change. I was great at trying to plow through changing the things that I could, but not so great at having the wisdom to know the difference. I was like the millions of other parents out there who feel that pull to show how super-human we are, because we think that is what folks want to see.

Forever searching for the silver lining, the positive within the difficult, I gradually began to learn that sometimes *there truly is no silver lining.* No happy ending or corner to be turned. What occurs is, rather, an internal shift. A backing up against the wall with one's higher power screaming, *Get out of your own way!*

I had to realize that perfect parenting did not exist. The inner and outer pressures to prove my worth as a mom needed to be quelled and replaced with a strong belief in what pediatric psychiatrist Donald Winnicott coined "good enough parenting" (Winnicott 1975, 237).

But the concept of "good enough" was hard for me to grasp. For someone who had lived her life serving others and seeking out perfection and goodness in the form of gold stars, it felt like learning a whole new language and worldview. Like *The Giving Tree*, I was lulled into soothing and helping everyone around me throughout my entire life. I had to begin to think of tending to my own needs as a counter-intuitive practice that would last a lifetime. But something had to change.

With deep trust that the universe would somehow have my back, I began to learn the value in letting go—into a liminal space of not knowing and not needing to control. The residual trauma of our son's orphanage experience that was now such a huge part of our lives was not of my own creation. Yet there I was, left to deal with its fallout.

I had to wonder, how was this different than other problems people incur that were not of their own making? Poverty. Hunger. Disease. War. Big questions loomed with no easy answers, other than giving a nod to the fact that life just sucks sometimes. Life isn't "fair," no matter how hard you try to spin what befalls you.

FOOD AND SUSTENANCE

I will never forget the first time I tried to feed Kai with a bottle. We were still in China. Because he was physically capable of eating solid food, our adoption social worker recommended bottle feeding to help facilitate the mother-child bond. He tolerated lying in my arms long enough to be fed when he was hungry, which nearly always was. Though Kai's cleft lip had been repaired, we knew even then that we'd need to get him surgery once we returned home. We had brought formula and squeezable cleft nursing bottles with us to China, but Kai was physically unable to suck or form a seal around the nipple of the bottle due to his poor oral muscle tone. Formula would drip along the sides of his face and down his chin, drenching his clothes and mine. By the end of the ordeal, Kai and I would both be covered in sweet, sticky formula. Thankfully, Scott kept Jade busy and engaged, offering to switch with me when he could tell that I needed a break.

I tried to use feeding time to connect and gaze into his eyes, and in turn, he would tightly squeeze them shut. While I knew full well he had suffered malnutrition, I was not prepared for the visceral reaction Kai would have to food and feeding. Like an animal, Kai lunged for food whenever it was in sight and raged when he couldn't have it. I couldn't believe what I was seeing—it felt very odd, sad and primitive.

Scott and Jade looked over curiously, while I explained to my daughter that Kai was just very, very hungry.

"Wow," Scott uttered, with an eyebrow raised curiously. "Do you remember those pictures we saw of Kai looking so skinny, Jade? Well, he didn't have anything in his tummy for much of the time. Can you imagine how it feels for him to get a full belly now? To have a family who will feed him whenever he is hungry?"

Kai's food gorging and hoarding made mealtimes extremely challenging. I truly saw the merit in Pavlov's research on involuntary reaction and response, having a child react so deeply and instinctively to seeing any type of food. It didn't matter what meal I prepared; Kai saw food and demanded to have it immediately, even foods that were not ready to eat, like raw meat.

We were always on edge, waiting for the next tantrum or control battle. The constant stress and conflict wore me down to a nub. Eventually, we learned that it was wise to put Kai down for a nap in his pack-and-play as I cooked, and Scott and Jade kept an eye on him. This way, we avoided the tantrums that inevitably ensued if he was unable to wait until we finished preparing dinner. We eventually called these tantrums "See-food tantrums," based on Kai's dynamic of throwing a complete fit if food was in his sight and he was unable to immediately have it. Having knowledge of reinforcement techniques, I knew that if I gave in to his violent tantrums and demands for us to instantly meet his needs, the tantrums would continue, so it was helpful to avoid this dynamic in the first place by timing food prep with nap time.

Kai even ate non-food items. One day, I looked over to the outdoor playset and was aghast to see our son sitting calmly at the bottom of the slide in his blue and green plaid shorts, sucking and chomping on a wood chip. I darted over, snatched it from his hand, and tossed it to the ground.

"What are you doing Kai? No! That's so yucky!" I exclaimed, looking him squarely in the eyes. He appeared to be unaffected, looking at me as if to say, "What's the problem here?" This was common.

Often he'd gnaw on grass and chew on sticks while playing in the backyard, until his watchful big sister would give us the heads up: "Mom, Dad, Kai's eating grass again." For the life of us, we couldn't understand this behavior, since he now had plenty to eat and could generally have it whenever he wanted. His urges seemed insatiable.

On one occasion, I turned away after putting a bowl of fruit salad on his highchair table, and he immediately grabbed two large grapes. His eyes widened as he stuffed both of them into his mouth at once. Bucking the chair in excitement, he grabbed more frantically, lunging toward the bread, crackers, and cold cuts on the table. I knew he would choke if I didn't sit with him and feed him one piece at a time, but we were late getting to the YMCA. I went to the fridge to get some milk, and by the time I returned to the table, Kai's eyes were bulging, his face was red, and he had gone quiet with his hands at his throat. I pulled off the highchair tray and started the Heimlich maneuver, pulling my clenched fists in toward his belly button. A half-eaten grape bolted out, and he was okay, thank God. Me? Not so much. I sank down to the wood kitchen floor and cried.

Sometimes, mealtimes ended in arguments between Scott and me. The tension around issues of food was palpable, made worse by the need to keep a sharp eye on Kai at all times. I knew that I was no longer a joy to be around. Hypervigilance was exhausting and I felt like a control freak, given really no option but to respond to my son's behaviors in the ways which I felt would keep him safe. The biological "mom sense"— an inability to tune out our children's behaviors—became a source of marital conflict because I was unable to ignore things that Scott could simply blow off.

For example, Kai's humming, tapping, thumping, and repetitive nonsense chatter drove me crazy. "What's that?" he would point to something he knew the answer to and wait for a response. At first, I'd respond with an answer, then another answer—until I began to feel like I was getting played. I got frustrated and angry. A therapist suggested reflecting these same questions back to him.

"I dunno Kai, *what IS that?*" While the technique helped, the constant noisemaking didn't stop.

Scott would ask, "Can't you just ignore him?"

"Seriously?" I'd respond. "No, I can't!"

While it's a huge generalization, I do think that women are wired to instinctively respond to the needs of others, especially children. Even if I could temporarily ignore the annoyances Kai would inflict upon the family, it didn't take long for the mounting, cumulative effect to eventually kick in. I tried to be empathic but ended up feeling like I was constantly trying to rein in my shit.

Despite giving us plenty of scares, Kai never actually did full-on choke. He did eat a yellowjacket though, on a sunny afternoon sitting at the little picnic table while inhaling his peanut butter and jelly sandwich. Similar to witnessing a train wreck in slow-motion, I watched in horror as the brightly colored insected landed on the edge of the sandwich crust just before it disappeared into his mouth. As I dashed over and attempted to pry his mouth open with my thumb and forefinger, Kai kicked and screamed, fighting against me

"Kai, you just ate a wasp! Open! Open!" I could see Kai had bitten the little bugger in half, the stinger firmly implanted in his tongue and still moving.

Despite the painful sting, Kai was dead set against relinquishing that chewed-up piece of PB and J from his mouth. Tears rolled down his face and he wailed, "Ow! Owie!"

"Kai, please don't fight me!" I retorted. "I want to get that wasp out of your mouth! Kai, open up. Stop fighting me!"

After about fifteen minutes and lots of tears, I finally pried his jaws apart and fished out the sludgy sandwich mixed with smeared yellow-jacket guts. From the little blood I could see, Kai had only been stung once, on his tongue, but it was hard to tell for sure. He did not swallow the thing (whew) and his breathing was not affected, but I watched him anxiously and intensely for the next couple of hours to see if he developed an allergic reaction. He did not, thankfully.

I thought to myself, *Wow. My son was so guarded against my taking food from his mouth, even as the wasp had the potential to really harm him.* Kai's instinctual desire to eat at all costs had almost had disastrous consequences.

At nap time, I cracked open a Corona and sat under the shade tree, breathing in deeply and shaking my head. I knew Kai harbored entrenched trauma and food concerns, but I had never conceived that these issues would potentially become dangerous, or fatal, if we didn't watch him closely 24/7. This constant fear added yet an additional tiresome layer to my already fraying nerves.

Kai's food issues morphed as he got older. Starting in kindergarten, we received regular phone calls from his teachers informing us he had stolen yet another student's snack or lunch, which often left his poor classmate in tears. Scott and I were constantly on the horn with teachers, brainstorming ways to address Kai's food insecurities while keeping the other kids' lunches safe. We were lucky to have had an amazing team of educators to work with, all of whom were open to being educated about orphanage trauma and neglect and its impact on a family or classroom.

Some families of children with food issues put locks on their cabinets. We did consider it for a brief time as a solution to food hoarding, but ultimately realized the need for locks was elsewhere. We ended up only locking the bathroom cabinet after discovering a large, empty bottle of mouthwash under Kai's bed one morning before he left for kindergarten. *Gahhh!* I screamed internally. I knew he tended to eat toothpaste, but this scared me. I had no idea what damage a child could do to his organs by drinking at least a half-bottle of Listerine. I called the poison control center to get advice. The nurse on the phone suggested that I keep a close eye on our little food ninja and to keep him home from school. The biggest concern was alcohol intoxication. Thankfully, he did not drink enough to become obliterated.

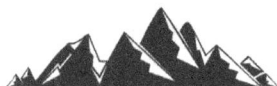

Comfort is a big deal, especially when one is feeling anxious or depressed and desperate to feel better somehow. Since Kai entered our life, I began to see food in ways I had never considered before. It's an entity which brings up intense feelings, such as safety, sustenance, and comfort, even for those denied food for a short term. Have you ever missed lunch and found yourself lashing out in hanger? Study upon study on the origins of addiction link the chemical dopamine to the positive feedback loop which satisfies a need for the immediate moment, only to repeat the cycle over and over again (Wise and Robble 2020).

For me, ice cream satisfies this chemical dopamine craving. I love me a Häagen-Dazs Caramel Cone Explosion sundae. Just thinking about eating one causes me to salivate, especially at the end of a long, hot summer day. I typically don't have ice cream in the house because I know I will eat the whole container in a day. When you continuously press the "More Dopamine" button in the feedback loop, these cravings become stronger and stronger. Some folks use alcohol or drugs. Others get their fix with technology. The mechanism is the same—craving, satisfaction, temporary relief, withdrawal. Then the cycle repeats itself.

Several years after Kai's food issues began banging around in my head, I began working as a hospital chaplain. While working on the medical floor, I met a woman who weighed over 500 pounds, who I'll call Kelly. Kelly was a hospital patient who had multiple comorbidities due to obesity, and little to no motivation to change. Staff avoided her because she acted surly and morose. They felt powerless in their efforts to help her, as she thwarted each caregiving attempt.

During our session, Kelly shared that she had experienced horrible physical and sexual abuse starting in the earliest years of her childhood. The men in her life "used her as a plaything," and food provided comfort to her when she felt unsafe. When she lacked control over her life, at least she could control her food. This pattern of consuming food to feel safe repeated itself as Kelly matured, until it was so firmly rooted that she was unable to change her relationship to food. Kelly admitted to me that she knew her weight jeopardized her health. As our conversation continued, she began to recognize that an unconscious motivation to gain more and more weight was to keep people away. The isolation she experienced sure beat feeling vulnerable and opening herself up to continued hurt feelings, which originated in her early years. She told me she appreciated that I risked asking her more about her past to understand her addiction to food, and I told her what I had learned from parenting Kai, in particular his relationship with food. She found our experience fascinating and could relate.

We talked a little about self-care, motherhood, and the conundrum women find ourselves in with the mixed messages we receive daily. Sure, we can care for ourselves, but there's always an expectation we sacrifice for our families. As our conversation wrapped up, she thanked me for feeling validated and seen. I felt grateful for having gained the knowledge I did from my son's experience, thankful that he had made progress in *his* healing, and appreciative that I could use the wisdom gained through my own private hell to help someone. I encouraged Kelly by acknowledging that it would not be easy. I admitted that trusting the process would be hard, yet assured her that making the decided effort to take better care of herself would definitely be worth it; *she* was worth it. As always, I needed to heed my own advice.

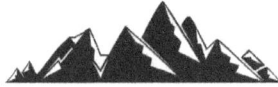

Kai's food issues waxed and waned as he got older, gradually subsiding. While it is always the hope to be done with the healing, it is a constant process. By the age of 13, his ever-present preoccupation with food eased a bit, and Scott, Jade and I breathed a sigh of relief that our diligent efforts to provide security and continuity had ultimately sunken in. Then, the COVID-19 pandemic hit, and again, we were all thrust into uncertainty. One morning early in the viral surge and accompanying lockdown, I discovered our cookie jar had mysteriously become depleted overnight. The following day, both full containers of blueberries and strawberries had disappeared. While not a huge deal in the grand scheme of things, I recognized that Kai's survival instinct (the need to hoard food) had returned, heightening our vigilance and family stress. Once again, we needed to regroup, reminding Kai that his need for safety is met here, and that he will always have enough food, even during a global pandemic.

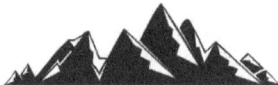

Still, the constant hypervigilance over his wellbeing felt agonizing. This was compounded by my fears of people judging me for poor parenting and my inability to be everywhere at all times. I worried about folks looking at me as if I was some kind of negligent parent who couldn't take good care of my child or blaming me that I "should have known" what I was getting into by adopting a child who had severe orphanage trauma. I questioned and re-thought everything through my retrospective guilt and shame-ridden lens of self-doubt.

This isn't how it should be, I thought to myself over and over again. Over time, my thinking switched to, *This is just how it is*. I plastered a fake smile upon my face and slogged through each day, searching for moments of reprieve, for hope and joy, for some message from the universe that I'd be okay.

UNDER WATER

When the kids were young, we joined the YMCA and I started working part-time as a swim instructor, which afforded us a discounted membership and classes for our kids. It was a great part-time gig, and we appreciated the strong sense of community focused around an active family lifestyle. The Y was terrific both for kids and for all four of us, giving us a place to recreate and have fun outside the home. The swimming pool proved to be a special treat for the kids, offering a zero-depth wading area, water features, and pool toys for heightened play and excitement.

We enrolled both Jade and Kai in swim lessons, realizing the importance of teaching them about all things aquatic. Water has its own way of teaching trust, among other lessons, in the natural realm: buoyancy, temperature, force, and movement. We were thrilled with Jade's enthusiasm as she moved up the class levels and embraced each new challenge, eventually joining the swim team. Often, she'd grab Kai's hand

and encourage him to jump in, but he consistently refused by plopping down on the pool deck, showing no interest in taking such risks.

Kai preferred sitting in one spot in the shallowest end of the wading pool. When he began lessons, Scott and I joked about inquiring if there was a "sea slug" level, as his temperament was one of exerting little-to-no effort with anything physical, much less an activity where he needed to keep himself afloat. At age four, he started at the toddler level with parent-child instruction, and I was grateful that his teacher had a patient-yet-firm temperament with him in the water.

While Kai loved sitting and splashing around in the water, swimming and floatation were completely different. As trust and interpersonal connection remained problematic, he would wiggle his slippery pudgy little body out of my arms, grunting with subtle disdain. Kai did not want to be held at all, much less in the water with near total skin-to-skin contact. Naturally, this can be an issue when a child doesn't know how to swim, so we would find ourselves becoming extra vigilant to keep him safe in the aquatic environment. He could not and would not comprehend the rationale of personal safety, so he needed to wear a floatation device at all times, which he surprisingly did not protest. Scott ultimately took my place in the parent-child swim class to give me a break, realizing that this could be a potential father-son bonding experience. Eventually, we gave up the idea of swimming lessons for him altogether, since Kai really showed no interest, and it was so much work to get him in the water. Even swimming—an activity which could have been fun—took on an unexpected arduousness.

I looked on with immense longing as I taught parent-tot swim lessons and noted the gleeful, affectionate interactions between the other moms and their toddlers, gazing into each other's eyes, gently nuzzling and trusting one another while learning to navigate buoyancy and floatation.

"Mom, catch me!" I would hear as I observed slithery, wet toddlers jumping into their parent's arms, giggling with confidence and elation.

There is such richness in the parent-child swim experience; I so yearned to have this with my son, but it was not yet possible.

My heart ached at the obviousness of my child's attachment challenges, while I watched typical, healthy parent-child interaction all around me. This was what I had expected and now felt deprived of with my son: deep, close, impactful experiences. I was pleased for the families in the classes I taught—they were living the family dream. This was exactly what I yearned for and why I wanted to parent—to intimately connect with my children in ways which were fun and exciting. Teaching parent-tot lessons accentuated the pain I felt as a new adoptive mom, and trying to teach my son on my own felt like a thwarted futile effort.

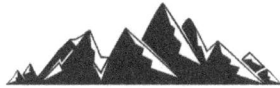

For years I continued to think, *If I just try hard enough, then…* (insert positive result), inevitably followed by, *It's not supposed to be like this.* Over time, I began to realize that parenting children through adoption was simply very different than biological parenting. Attachment style is on a spectrum, and some foster and adoptive children struggle more than others. Accepting this fact was paramount to my wellbeing and the wellbeing of our family.

The drudgery of parenting Kai brought us down, and Scott and I began to argue with the least amount of provocation. Children with histories of trauma frequently create chaos and split with their caregivers because it gives them a feeling of control and mastery over the interpersonal dynamics. For example, when Kai would feign ignorance about some knowledge or skill he had acquired, I held him accountable. Snapping himself into and out of his car seat, for instance, was something he was completely able to do, yet he preferred to let Dad perform this task over and over again. One day, I blew up at Scott in exasperation.

"He's totally manipulating you, Scott," I said. "He's got you sucked into doing it for him and he's secretly hoping we argue about it."

Over the years, I learned that Kai's abilities were his best kept secret, concealed under learned helplessness, behavioral problems, and what felt like his tendency to work the system, including Scott's and my marriage.

Of course, these dynamics wove their way into Kai's school days, and it predictably took a couple of months for teachers to catch on, year after year. It was frustrating at best, maddening at worst. Over time, Scott and I learned to get on the same page and to communicate with his teachers. We learned to *expect* challenges, and for Kai to thwart my efforts and the efforts of his teachers to help him. It was mentally taxing, hard, and draining work.

We desperately needed fun in our lives. We craved adventure. We began to think about how we could uniquely embrace who we were in ways that brought us strength and joy, piggybacking upon the shared interests that brought Scott and I together, as joy and adventure had once been the backbone of our marriage. Now that we were responsible adults (and parents, of course), we knew smoking pot and drinking ourselves into oblivion weren't viable options for coping with the stress (one of the drawbacks of having two folks with mental health backgrounds—knowledge of the slippery slope).

Our desires for fun and adventure were hobbled by the daily grind, and by the reality that we existed in a perpetual crisis mode, day after day. The best I could do was to squeeze in moments of self-care whenever I could, plan for the annual family vacay, and hope to rekindle a sense of purpose and joy. I'd felt that I lost myself, in a sense. And I wanted to find her.

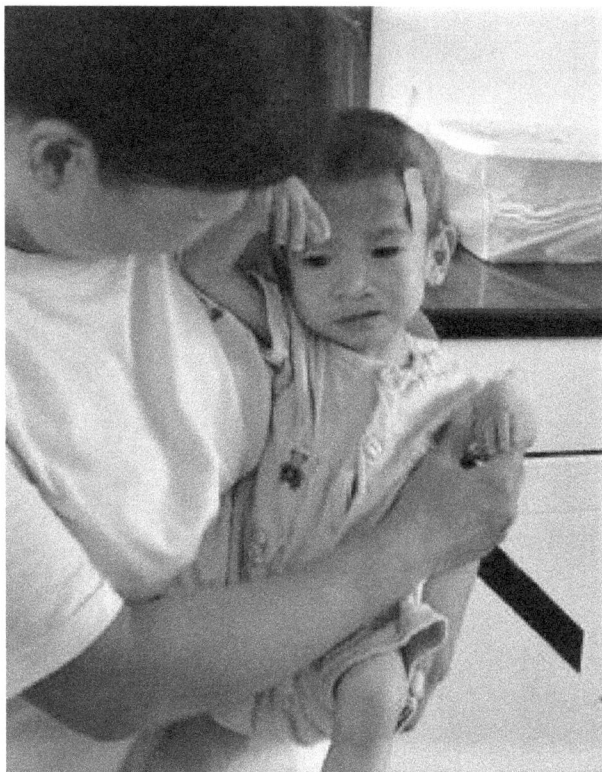

Pre-adoption, at the orphanage, 2007.

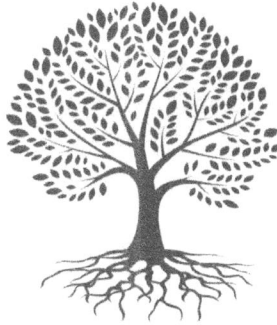

CHAPTER 2

BROKEN BODY, BROKEN PRIDE

My son's therapist warned me that I was on the road to burnout, but I didn't believe him. I was dead set on proving that my mama-bear strength and tenacity would carry us through.

Parenting a child with a history of trauma isn't for the fainthearted. I'd venture to say that, for most people, it isn't well understood either, as most of us tend to generalize that parent-child attachment is normal, children are resilient, and parent-child bonding happens naturally. Sometimes this isn't the case.

The unfortunate truth is that children from institutions often harbor an unconscious fear of being forgotten. Hence, they create constant noise in the form of incessant nonsense chatter, thumping, humming, tapping, or other maddening "under the radar" ways to remain in your awareness. I often describe it as "death by a thousand cuts." When you live with constant random noise, a never ending twitchy hyper-alertness permeates the entire family unit—usually felt most intensely by the primary caregiver. Living this way for an extended time creates a kind of chronic post-traumatic stress. Since we're wired to respond to our children, these children develop a knack for finding the last nerve you've got and playing it like a fiddle.

On one particular night, on a February evening when Kai was in first grade, I heard a loud noise around 10:30pm. From the other side of our bedroom wall I heard, *thump, thump. Thump.* Scott had work in the morning and the kids had school. This was not the time for noise-making. *Thump.*

"He's bumping the wall again," I said to Scott, who is the heaviest sleeper I have ever known. The kids and I have always joked that he has the ability to fall asleep standing up in a hurricane.

"What? Huh? Ugh. I was sleeping," he said.

Jade heard the thumping and came into our room. "Mom, can you tell Kai to stop? I can't sleep."

I ambled over to his bedroom and creaked open the door. Kai looked at me and smirked, as if he was proud to be keeping us up. I laid into him. "Kai go to sleep! Stop thumping! We need rest!"

As if he sensed my anger was some kind of badge of personal honor, he continued hitting the wall, louder and louder. Even after I returned to my room, the *thump*ing didn't stop. Jade was tired. My last nerve was frayed and I was livid. I was also thankful that he was still small enough to carry.

It was midnight, and we only had six potential hours left of sleep. I stomped back over to his bedroom after multiple warnings for him to stop. I blasted open the door, walked over to his bed, picked him up in his red blanket sleeper and threw him over my hip. Kai was laughing. He didn't fight me as I carried him downstairs, pretending to feel calm. I walked to the sliding glass doors leading to the deck and opened them. There was a nice, packed snowbank as tall as my knees. Inwardly laughing to myself for feeling like a fed-up, horrible mom, I extended my arms with Kai in tow and plopped him into the snowbank. His eyes widened as he looked up at me, surprised that I would do such a thing.

"Are you done *thump*ing?" I probed.

He nodded his head, eyebrows raised in incredulity. I was surprised he didn't fuss. It was like he knew he needed this kind of action to jolt him into awareness that I was serious. Something in me was aware that Kai *knew* he was being a little shit. I helped him dust the snow off his pajamas and led him by the hand back upstairs to his bedroom. He climbed back into his toddler bed, and we all slept soundly, at last.

But this wasn't a one-time problem. Another night, I made a nice family dinner, complete with salmon, rice, and salad. Kai was in middle school. We were all sitting at the table talking about our days, when suddenly to my right, I heard him smacking his food in his mouth: *smack, smack, smack.* I turned to him and asked politely, "Kai, please stop your smacking." He persisted. *Smack. Smack.* I reminded him that it's gross. "Kai, that's disgusting. No one wants to see your food."

He continued *smack*ing, with no concern nor care about how this impacted those at the table. I had learned to let it go, yet my anger continued to simmer just under the surface. I knew this kid didn't care. And he didn't care that *we did*.

In time, I began to realize that a "dull hum" of irritation, as I often referred to it, had permeated my existence. I was silently trying to go about my life, trying to not allow these constant, mounting irritations to get to me and knowing my daughter was trying to do the same.

Scott asked, "Can't you just ignore him?" This fueled my angst because the annoyances felt nonstop. Kai saved this objectionable behavior for me and Jade in a way that felt brilliantly calculated. Even if I could have ignored him, my heartrate was elevated from my utter exasperation. I felt depleted and bone tired. Deep down, I knew that these behaviors were probably unconscious, but that knowledge didn't make living with them any easier. I felt a tension between wanting to share what I was going through and an expectation to keep it to myself.

These small daily assaults on my wellbeing were beginning to take their toll, and I felt stuck.

TRAUMA BEGETS TRAUMA

I can be amazingly headstrong and stubborn; sometimes these qualities come in handy and sometimes they become problematic. They're great when I've got a goal in mind, when I need to break into mama-bear mode for my children, or when I'm in professional situations requiring quick, confident decision making. Yet when parenting a child of trauma, all bets are off. Previous understandings about parenting and nurturing are useless. Well-intentioned efforts to help are stymied. Tenacity, resolve, and determination, all qualities I had always prided myself in, are thwarted. All attributes of personal power and efficacy shift to the wayside as the reality of your child's unresolved trauma breaks to the surface.

As Kai's needs increased and parental pressures in our home mounted, my felt desire to prove my worthiness as a mom also grew. I had never considered that adoptive parenting would create such feelings of inadequacy within me. These difficult emotions came in stark comparison to the "normal" emotions I'd expected to feel while parenting a "normal" child. But this situation was a different reality, and a decidedly complex one at that. I continued to draw upon my energy reserves nonetheless, exerting one hundred percent of my effort, day after day, to raise my children.

As time marched on and Kai's development appeared to move slower than a snail's pace, I turned to the myriad services available to help him, because I knew I couldn't do it all. We were able to access occupational, physical, and speech therapy through our state's Birth-to-Three program, which is a publicly funded early intervention special education service. Kai began eligibility testing and underwent a plethora of exams to determine why he had so many delays and behavioral problems. For over a year, extensive medical workups of one sort or another dominated our lives. Assessments of his endocrinology, neuropsychology, and genetics were done alongside MRIs and interventional radiological testing. Evaluation after evaluation came back inconclusive, resulting in head-scratching for all involved, including Kai's medical team. He was a complex kid with no definitive etiology for his problems or symptoms, other than a substantial history of profound orphanage neglect and developmental trauma.

This experience was a complete contrast with our daughter's development, which felt much more typical, enjoyable, and engaging. Scott and I began to worry about our emotional and financial resources, as many of these new needs required specialists outside of our insurance network. It felt like we never had enough money or emotional reserves, yet we kept forging ahead in pursuit of whatever could help our son.

I had hoped to gain a sense of encouragement, a lightened heart, and a clearer mind, but those weren't forthcoming. What I had begun to feel was an immense sense of responsibility, never-ending toil, and pervasive heartache that I feared would never end.

"Your son is very delayed," one specialist shared. "These problems seldom resolve themselves since these children's brains are formed in such neglectful circumstances. It's not that they don't *want* to attach. They *can't*. Those neuropathways wired to seek out connection, nurture, and learning will always be impacted, as if your child has a brain injury. If you look at PET scans of these kids' brains, you'll see it. With typically developing children, the areas of the brain connected with learning and nurture light up. With kids with such profound institutional neglect like Kai, they're dark. It's really, really sad."

I kept thinking, *We're educated in these things. Can I work harder? No. I'm already coming apart at the seams.* We weren't able to get a PET scan for our son, but each specialist concurred that the etiology (the medical term for "cause") of our son's problems was orphanage neglect. His lack of early nurture contributed to a type of disconnect that would take years to heal—if at all. I wondered, *How will the days ahead ensue? How will I survive? How will we survive?*

From the moment my eyes opened in the morning until they closed at night, I slogged through, trying to sneak in as many valuable learning experiences for the kids as I could, while attempting to move the process along as quickly as possible. Like my strong German grandma trying to get me to eat the gross potato salad that she was sure would heal whatever ailed me, I was stubbornly determined to make my child well.

CRASHING DOWN

My body has always been my ally. As far back as I can remember, I found solace by tramping barefoot in the outdoors, feeling the warm sun beaming down on my freshly tanned, dirt-patinaed skin, and running around the neighborhood from dusk to dawn. Like many athletes, I find movement integral to my wellbeing. When I'm stressed or in a bad headspace, the fluid movement of climbing (requiring intense "in the moment" concentration) propels me into a better frame of mind, where the worries of the day are left in the dust.

I inherited my dad's athletic constitution, with formidable mind-body awareness and natural sense of strength, which lent itself to all kinds of sports. My dad was well-known in the small town where I grew up as a remarkably gifted athlete. He was a softball hall-of-famer, known as the guy to win the game by hitting the ball over the fence. He turned to the milder game of golf in his later years. Even well into his 70s, his tee-off was like a shot out of a cannon, and he continued to be a "force on the course," gaining newspaper acclaim for a hole-in-one and the occasional noteworthy senior tournament score.

As I grew older, I gained a greater understanding of how I was like my father and how important movement is to my overall wellbeing.

After long periods of sitting, my thinking would become sludgy, cluttered, and dim, bordering on clinical depression. Movement for me was like an oil change. It cleared thoughts and allowed my mind to run smoothly. All worries and concerns dissipated after a mental detox in the form of intense exercise.

Rock-climbing was a gritty, intense, *all-in* mind-body outdoor activity that held an edginess and an element of thrill-seeking that Scott and I embraced with both arms. We turned rock-climbing into a family affair once the kids came along.

In the fall of 2011, Jade was in first grade, Kai was in morning kindergarten, and Scott was working in a school. In addition, Kai had therapy appointments daily and sessions with various specialists scheduled throughout the week, so I needed to squeeze in my own need for exercise or self-care whenever extra time was available. Schlepping Kai along with me to the gym, I would pack up a bag with ancillary toys, board books, and matchbox cars to keep him occupied while I carved out a little time to get my climb on. It was important for me to find these moments of temporary reprieve from my parenting stress.

Driving to the climbing gym, I went through my mental checklist of all the things I needed to do during the day. Appointment with pediatrician later in the afternoon—*check*. Bag of belongings—*check*. Kai's medication list—*check*. Baggie of Cheez-Its for Kai to snack on— *check*. I parked my car in the lot and ran around the car to get Kai out of his seat, questioning if there was anything I had forgotten. It had become routine to think several steps ahead before leaving the house, but I always wondered if I had forgotten some important detail.

I checked in with a coworker at the front desk. "Hey Alex, lots going on today. I'll be doing some speed climbing. Need to be outta here by two."

"Hey, sounds good!" he responded. "We've got some cool new routes set up; check 'em out!"

I donned my climbing harness, chalk bag, and shoes, and set Kai up with his matchbox cars on the carpeted gym floor in a central place where I could keep an eye on him. He wasn't one to move around much, and there were times I was actually thankful for this—I could set him up somewhere with his toys and he would stay put. We noted often that Kai's tendency to ooze into a zoned-out lump on the floor—while not optimal—was occasionally handy. Knowing my time was limited, I hopped on a few auto belays, ropes that allow for independent climbing, to warm up before striking up a conversation about the enticing new routes with some other climbing friends. I briefly glanced over at Kai, who was laying on his side, running the wheels of a car along the cover of a book again and again. He held his work close to his face, his little tongue poking out of the corner of his mouth in concentration. *I should probably snag those Cheez-Its before he dumps them on the floor, or even worse—chokes on them,* I thought. *Oh, and I should probably call Scott about dinner tonight, since I'll be home late. Shoot.* I looked back at my friend. Could she tell I was thinking of other things besides the climbing wall in front of me? I felt as if a continuous revving motor ran in my brain. This was just the way it was these days.

"Kai, stop lining up your cars," I called. "Quit spinning the car wheels and let's do some pretend play." I felt a need to constantly redirect Kai's attention to some new stimulation, since his inclination was to completely zone out. It is almost impossible to turn this "mom sense" off, despite knowing the importance of doing so sometimes. We're just always on—with our finely tuned, sensitive mom radar stuck in hyperaware mode. I was, without question, operating in unacknowledged, full-on burnout mode, masquerading as super-mom.

I turned back to the fun, new route set up on the first wall to my left, with small crimpy climbing holds. Climbing this would require some good, challenging moves.

"What's the rating on this one?" I asked Alex, as it did not have a difficulty rating number posted.

"Not sure," he called back. "I can't remember who set it. Looks like maybe a moderate 5.10? 5.10 minus?" I liked the way the route started to the left of the corner, with dynamic, creative moves going around to the right as it got to the top.

"Sweet," I shouted back, darting back over to the wall from across the gym. As I nearly reached the top, my hand slipped off the sloping hold, but I didn't feel the "catch" of the rope on my harness. *Shit!* I had forgotten to clip in—I was falling.

Dammit! Oh my God! I fucking forgot to clip in!

My body plunged 30 feet, crashing on the carpeted gym floor with my dominant right leg leading. On reflex, I attempted to get up to let everyone know I was fine—my brain had not caught up with the reality that I had shattered my pelvis, vertebra, and ankle. My body collapsed back on to the floor like a rag doll. *My God. How could I have done this?!* I exclaimed to myself, a thought so loud I'm certain everyone around me heard. *How could I have let my pent-up stress cloud my judgement this badly? How could I have made such a horrible mistake? Shit!*

Kai was still playing nearby as the gym manager Greg rushed over to tend to my crumbled heap of a body. In shock, I lamented to Greg and myself, over and over, "Oh my God, I'm so sorry. Fuckin'A! what the hell? I knew better. Shit! I totally fucked up!"

"Don't worry about it, Chris. It happened," Greg replied. "Just try to stay still. We called the paramedics, and they're on their way." He continued to hold the base of my head and neck in place in anticipation of the arrival of the paramedics. I wondered, *Why is he holding my neck? Does he think I have a spinal cord injury? I landed feet first. Something's off with my lower back and hips. Shit. Something's not connected there. Fuck.*

As we waited for the ambulance to arrive and the comforting aura of shock continued to protect me, the intense stress I had been living in came bursting back into my awareness with greater and greater intensity. I had fucked up my body. It was too late to turn back.

Shattered and broken on the floor, I knew I could not hit rewind. I would need to face the complex clusterfuck I had been trying to conceal—the presumed "okayness" with the daily dread, the loneliness, the isolation—now accompanied by feelings of hurt, resentment, and terror which came oozing out of my consciousness, along with the blood from the huge gash in my upper lip.

Tears seeped out the corners of my eyes as anger at myself crept in, along with horror at what had just transpired, and I uttered obscenity after obscenity to express my pent-up frustration and complete exhaustion. "Shit! I have been *so fucking stressed!* Dammit! How could I let this happen?! *Fuuckk!*" The armor of my pride shattered the instant I hit the floor and now exposed my vulnerable and tender, broken spirit.

I realized I had bitten through my upper lip on impact, leaving a bloodied hunk of skin hanging as I continued to speak, which I desperately had the urge to bite off but had the presence of mind not to. Greg continued to hold my head and neck in place as a precautionary move, assuring me that the ambulance was coming. In my angst-ridden state, all I could do was continue releasing strings of obscenities.

"Greg, you have no fucking clue how hard it's been. Shit! This kid— oh, my God. *Uggg—I'm so Goddamn fucking pissed!*" Suddenly, my mind rebounded into mom-mode.

"Kai is supposed to be at an appointment at 3:00 with Dr. North! Can someone call the office to let them know we won't be there? The number is in my phone. And can someone call Scott at work?"

"Sure, Chris," Greg assured. "I think we have his number in the system."

"Be sure to hit extension 175 or you'll go directly to the secretary," I suggested.

"I can't believe you're even with-it enough to tell us this stuff," someone uttered from a few feet behind me. I became aware that a small crowd had assembled, looking on with concern. I thought to myself, *This probably seems pretty messed up—autopilot mom-mode is still in full swing.*

Alex assured me that the trusted gym staff was caring for Kai in the back room. As he talked, what had happened gradually began seeping back into my awareness, along with a burning, searing pain that was now starting to rush into my broken body.

The paramedics arrived within ten minutes and promptly cut off my climbing harness and right shoe, while agonizing pain ballooned in my swollen, misshapen ankle. Two tan, athletic-looking guys hooked up an IV and stuck the needle in my arm, allowing a welcome drip of narcotics to quell both my mounting pain and my increasing anxiety. As they fastened a cervical collar around my neck and slid me onto a backboard, it became clear to me that something wasn't right. I felt eerily like a marionette at the base of my pelvis, where the bones had obviously disconnected from each other. Just as my fear was mounting, the pain medicine took over, finally letting me chill out and let the medical folks handle the situation. For the first time since I can remember, I let go of my need to control and trusted other people. I released my grip on the outcome because I had to. *My God,* I thought, *thank God for modern medicine.* I began to allow myself to ease into the calm of whatever IV pain meds had thankfully taken effect.

BROKEN

As the ambulance pulled away and the siren began to howl, I thought about my son whom I had left behind. I wondered what he had witnessed, how much he took in, and if he even caught on to the seriousness of the entire ordeal. Part of me doubted that he understood, since he was usually in a world of his own—lining up his matchbox cars or perseverating on the spinning wheels. I felt a constant need to pull his attention and awareness into the present. Now, ironically, I was the one who had not been present, and it had cost me so, so dearly. My constant focus on the actions and needs of others had caused me to suffer the consequences of being so completely distracted. My the reality of my utter inattention to myself—to my own safety and wellbeing—crashed down into my awareness.

Feeling an odd combination of dread mixed with somber, quiet relief, I admitted to the paramedic sitting beside me, "You know, in an odd way, I probably needed something like this to happen. I was parenting on overdrive, in constant stress and burnout mode. I didn't do this on purpose, but *something* had to give."

He acknowledged that parenting can definitely be challenging. "There's a saying among paramedics: 'That's why we call them accidents.'"

The previous week, I had squeezed in an hour to buy myself a workout outfit and found a cute, peach-colored, moisture-wicking, sleeveless top and a perfect-fitting pair of gray yoga pants. Deliberating over whether I should spend the money on myself, I had thought, *Why not?* I felt good in them. The pants were long enough, which was a rarity for my long legs. I wasn't sure if or when I'd have time to shop for myself again in the foreseeable future.

Now, my clothing was stained from the blood that dripped down from my chomped lip. It didn't matter. The drugs dampened any concerns I had, at least somewhat, at least for now.

At the hospital, I watched with interest and amazement as the emergency room personnel lost no time in assessing the extent of my injuries. The medical team slid my body onto something called a "hover mat," and a nurse procured a large pair of scissors to cut down the center of my clothing.

"Sorry about this," a young brunette nurse said. "It's just something we have to do."

I watched with feelings of dismay and embarrassment as she proceeded to snip down the middle of my brand-new shirt and the sides of my perfect-fitting gray yoga pants.

This clothing symbolized my freedom and mobility, my pride in my abilities, and my sense of self, which I now observed being ripped apart and discarded without hesitation. Waves of sadness and bitter disappointment rushed in while the hustle continued. I looked on in disbelief and utter defeat as these beloved garments were hastily tossed into a garbage bag in the corner of the room. Like crumbled, fallen autumn leaves who had served their purpose, they were now part of the ash-heap.

I choked back the tears and decided to channel my attention toward my fascination with what was happening around me in the trauma bay. The rush of heightened activity and sense of urgency piqued my curiosity, as my naked, broken body lay exposed and cold.

Feeling embarrassed, powerless, and raw, I looked around the room at the ubiquitous white walls and stainless steel appliances. An antiseptic smell filled the air, and I peered at the white-tiled ceiling, trying hard to maintain my integrity and sense of okay-ness, which was beginning to dissipate. I looked up at the IV medication bag attached to my arm, comforted by the clicking that reassured me the drugs were steadily being released and doing their thing.

"Let me get you a warm blanket," the kind nurse offered, seeming to be aware that the hospital staff were all in complete "action" mode, treating my sense of comfort was a fleeting yet important afterthought. "Sorry, we keep it pretty cold in here." She also reassured me that she could remove my C-collar, since they weren't worried about a spinal cord injury.

"That would be great," I responded, not clear if my shivering was due to the chill in the air or the fact that I was in shock. When the warm, heated blanket arrived and this sweet caring nurse placed it over me, it felt calming nonetheless.

I encouraged myself to ride the wave of pain meds and allow them to lull my monkey-mind into quiet and peaceful passivity. I wanted to get out of my thinking, solving brain and embrace a calming sense of trust. This non-negotiable acceptance of care and concern was the antithesis of my nature, yet I knew I had no choice. More and more realizations about my broken body came to me in waves.

My pelvis is not connected. My ankle is pounding, contorted, and swelling like a balloon. My lip is dangling over my teeth—I want to bite the dang thing off! My nose hurts. I see it swelling—I must have kneed myself in the face on impact. The knuckles on my right hand are scraped and bleeding. Did I try to grab a bolt or a quickdraw on the way down? I must have. God, with my lip dangling down and blood all over my face, I must look completely hideous. I want this to be over. I want my life back. Shit. I was off the hook from parenting, but this was a sucky alternative.

It was like an unrelenting emotional downpour, with no end in sight. I never lost consciousness, which is a good thing. There was no brain injury and not enough internal damage or blood loss for the body to shut itself down. I wouldn't die from my injuries—promising news.

As I was taken by a hospital transporter for CT scans, X-rays, and ultrasounds, I peppered staff with questions, which they obviously could not answer. I wanted reassurance that everything would be okay, that my injuries were manageable and no big deal, which was clearly not the case. I wished so hard that I could undo the accident, that I could revisit the moment I forgot to clip into the damned auto belay.

Scott finally arrived at the emergency department. Pulling aside the light green plaid curtain, he poked his head around the corner and peered at me with a combination of curiosity and grave concern. Our eyes locked, and I fought back my usual inclination to downplay the direness of the circumstances.

"I'd kiss you," Scott said, "but it looks like you've done a number on your lip. Oh my God, Chris, I was worried sick." He took off his denim jacket and plaid scarf and sat down beside me.

"I must look like shit," I said, trying to curb the seriousness of the situation he was now seeing me in. Both of us are the type to "tough it out." We want to minimize situations of difficulty for the purpose of soldiering on, to eschew dependency or neediness in favor of self-reliance and physical and emotional fortitude. The obviousness of my condition took some time to register, and the look on Scott's face showed me he was not prepared for what he was seeing. Our modus operandi—the way we typically took on the world as a couple—was about to be challenged. Neither of us knew how to do this. "Life adventure" would come to take on a whole new meaning.

"I got to the climbing gym just as the ambulance pulled out of the parking lot," Scott said. "Sarah from the front desk called me at work and had to have me paged. That never happens. She mentioned you'd had a pretty bad fall, but when she said, 'She's still with us,' my mind went to all sorts of bad places."

I filled him in on what happened. As he leaned toward me and grabbed my hand, he commented on my bloodied knuckles, which he also thought was from trying to grab the quickdraws on the wall during my fall. "Oh my God, Chris. I was so worried. I really thought you had almost died. I couldn't get that out of my head until now."

"Really?" I asked. "They thought I was that bad?" I was still trying hard to minimize what had happened to me, secretly hoping that my denial would win out and that this would all dissipate as a horrible, bad dream.

"Where are the kids?" I asked.

"My mom is picking Jade up at school—I called school to let staff know, and of course they're concerned. The gym is keeping Kai until Mom is able to get him. Then, Mom and the kids will come here, in about an hour or so, I think," he replied. "I think she'll keep them in the waiting room."

Reflexively, my mom-sense kicked in and I wondered out loud whether Kai's behavior would be problematic in the waiting room. I envisioned him grabbing other peoples' snacks and whining, causing problems for Scott's mom and the desk staff.

"Oh my God, Chris, don't worry about it," Scott responded. "You really just need to focus on yourself right now. My mom's got this. Relax."

"You know, all the stress we've been under contributed to this," I said. "Seriously, all the stress of parenting Kai. The hypervigilance. Feeling constantly wound up tight. It finally caught up with me, Scott."

Scott sighed and looked down at the ground briefly, before peering back at me. "Yeah, I don't doubt that. Let's just what see what the doctor has to say. We need to keep the focus on you now."

The resident orthopedic surgeon appeared shortly afterward, with his young entourage of medical students in tow. He extended his hand to introduce himself, as the white-jacketed crew accompanying him looked at me and then back at him, eager for this next learning opportunity. Scott stood up and walked into the corner beside me, holding my hand as he braced for whatever news would be forthcoming.

"Well, we have a few things going on," the resident began. He pulled up my X-rays and CT scans on the computer.

"We'll start with your back. You've fractured a few vertebra—your L1, L4, and L5. I think with a brace, those will eventually heal on their own. Now for the more concerning stuff. You broke your pelvis—the ring that supports your spine and the rest of your body. We call this kind of fracture a 'vertical shear' pelvic ring fracture, and these are very serious. I'm pleasantly surprised that you avoided additional organ damage, and the ultrasounds and CT scans seem to show that everything is okay. Your kidneys, bladder: all are intact with no internal bleeding. But the right side of your pelvic ring will need to be brought back down and surgically realigned."

On the X-rays, my ankle looked like a piece of pottery that had been smashed to smithereens. My pelvic ring had broken in half, and my sacrum—the hearty "V" shaped bone at the bottom of the spine connected to both hips—looked like a sheared teacup. My rami—the "sitting bones" at the bottom of my pelvis—were not connected.

The three-dimensional CT scan of my ankle looked like a jagged, hollowed-out tree trunk. None of it looked good.

"So, what does all this mean?" I asked. "Are you saying I'll be admitted to the hospital?" My denial was an ocean deep. I so desperately wanted to believe that life would go on as it had before. Before the accident. Before everything came crashing down.

The nurses, the doctor and the medical students glanced at each other with raised eyebrows while the resident spoke. "Oh, you'll be in the hospital for a while. Your injuries are pretty severe."

I'd only ever had one other experience with being in the hospital: in fifth grade, I had to get three stitches after hitting my shin on the pool deck.

The resident surgeon continued his explanation. "We will need to put your leg into traction for a couple of days to pull it back into position before surgery, so in a few minutes we'll have to drill a pin through your femur before you go up to the medical floor. There, they'll set up a frame with a 20-pound weight to pull your leg back down."

"Wait—" I gasped. "You're gonna drill through my leg? Like, right here?" The students and nurses inhaled, as if they had anticipated my reaction.

"Yes," the resident said. "We can give you something to take the edge off. It won't take long. The nurse and your husband can hold your hand. It'll go quick."

Scott and I stared at each other, squeezing one another's hands as we readied for the next round of news.

"I think I'm gonna sit back down for now, if that's okay with you," Scott said.

"Of course," I responded and released my grip. "This is so much to take in."

"I know it is," the doctor replied. "It is a lot. You got very badly hurt."

I wanted to know what to expect in the days and years ahead. *Would I be in constant pain? Would I walk normally again? Would there be potential complications?* I kept these questions to myself as I let the doctor continue with his discourse. I thanked my lucky stars for the pain medication, which was obviously continuing to do its job, since I was learning just how serious my injuries were but not yet feeling them.

"Now for your ankle. Chris, you basically destroyed your ankle. You shattered it. These kinds of fractures—we call them 'pilon' or 'tibial plafond' fractures—are notoriously hard to fix. Potential complications include post-traumatic arthritis, fracture blisters and skin breakdown, the need for additional future surgeries—including plastic surgery, amputation—"

"Wait!" I interrupted. "*Amputation?* Seriously?"

The resident surgeon leaned against the foot of my bed, conveying that this was not a typical "smack on a cast and let it heal" fracture. This was a life-altering injury that would require lots of deliberating, reassessing, and hand-wringing. He proceeded to express his utmost confidence in the skills of his attending orthopedic surgeon, who I would meet two days later in the operating room.

I looked at Scott, his face now showing a light sheen of perspiration. "Is it getting hot in here, or is it just me?" He took off the next layer of clothing, a blue and white Nordic-style sweater.

"Do you have any more questions?" the doctor asked.

Too many questions swirled around in my head, and I was too overwhelmed to even address them. I knew that I would need time to let all of this information sink in but wondered if I would have the time to let it catch up to me. The team assured me they would be back shortly, then filed out of the room.

"Amputation?" I turned to Scott.

"Chris, you know they have to give you the worst-case scenario. It's part of their jobs."

A nurse came back in to check on us and briefly glanced over at Scott, who sat with his head back against the wall, sans sweater, in a Fruit-of-the-Loom undershirt, looking pallid.

"Uh-oh," the nurse said, backing out of the room momentarily and signaling for one of her colleagues. "He's not looking too well."

"Whaddaya mean?" I replied, now seeing that Scott was on the verge of passing out.

"I think we will need to take him next door and make him a quick patient," she said. "We see this a lot with overwhelmed spouses. Mostly the men." The nurse winked at me and pulled in the gurney that her partner had delivered.

Scott continued to press his head against the wall, acknowledging he was out of sorts.

"So much for my knight in shining armor," I said.

The nurses and I chuckled as they assisted him on to the rolling gurney and rolled him out the door, saying they would give him lots of apple juice and water while monitoring his vitals.

The medical crew returned with a small drill in hand. My nurse added what was very likely Valium or some other nerve-soothing medication to my IV before walking around to the right side of my bed.

"Do you think you're ready?" she asked.

"Hell no. Do I have a choice though?" We both laughed, accepting that I did not.

She held my hand as the resident and his entourage attached a narrow stainless-steel bit to the drill before boring through my tender flesh, just above my knee.

"I don't think I'd watch if I were you," she advised, putting her other warm hand on my shoulder.

"No, I don't think I will. I'll just close my eyes and grit my teeth until it's over."

"Good idea. I will too," she answered, squeezing my hand as the high-pitched drilling began—and dug through one side of my femur to the other. I squeezed my eyes shut as the sparkling silver drill bit burrowed through my skin and bone. Searing pain registered in my brain as I fought hard to hold back the tears, acutely aware that the pain and anxiety meds were thankfully tempering the agony a bit. My thigh felt hot. My entire leg throbbed.

I looked up at the nurse beside my bed when the drilling stopped. One tear leaked out of my left eye, and I asked, "Are we done?"

"Yes," she said, squeezing my hand more tightly before gently touching my shoulder. "You did great. You must have nerves of steel because most people don't do so well. Congrats."

I was informed that the staff would continue to look after Scott, and he would be sent home.

"Sorry," my nurse apologized. "He became a patient when he started passing out. He'll be discharged home with your mother-in-law, and she assured me that your kids are doing okay. They can see you on the medical floor tomorrow." I felt torn between disappointment that I couldn't see my family and relief that I could finally drift off and have time alone, at last.

PEACE, QUIET, AND STILLNESS

I got to my hospital room on the trauma floor right around dusk. The setting sun peered through the tinted window and half-pulled shade, gleaming across the floor and onto the starched white blankets covering my body. A man carrying clanking metal hardware and long metal bars came into the room and introduced himself.

"I'm here to set up your traction. I might be a little loud, but it shouldn't take long."

Everything about the way this all worked was so interesting! I watched with curiosity and talked with him as he screwed the long, angled metal contraption to my bed, before staff returned with the 20-pound weight to hang off the end. The weight was attached to a pulley system on the metal structure, which was attached to my leg. With it, they suspended my leg above the bed so that my pelvic bones would be held in proper alignment. A triangle hanging bar hung just above my head, and I was told I could use it to hoist myself up. I joked that I'd use it for practicing gymnastics and that I'd work on perfecting my dismount.

After the sun set and the room became dark, a peaceful hush blanketed me, bringing an odd sense of serenity and relief.

Maybe it's the pain meds, I thought to myself.

But no, the calm I felt had a lot more to do with the weight that had just been lifted off my shoulders—the weight of parenting a child of trauma, and the pent-up angst I had been carrying around like a pressure-cooker, waiting to burst.

A warm, salty tear rolled down my cheek as the gravity of the situation began to permeate my awareness—the stress of parenting as well as the seriousness of my injuries. I closed my eyes, took a deep breath, and finally, exhaled myself off the parenting hook. For the foreseeable future, my job would be to focus on my own healing—an all-encompassing endeavor.

Perhaps for the first time ever, my entrenched sense of pride in my abilities, inner strength and outer fortitude, and tendencies toward uber-responsibility were replaced with a much-needed reprieve. Now, a mandatory emotional, physical, and spiritual time-out was on the horizon, with the elusive promise of healing somewhere in the cosmos.

I peered at the shadow on the wall of the gently swaying branches from the willow tree outside my window. The last bold orange rays from the setting sun flickered into the corner of the room. A blanket of calm overcame me as I watched a solitary dry leaf flap in the wind, clinging to the tree's waving branch with all her might. She let go and gently floated downward with the breeze. I drifted off to sleep.

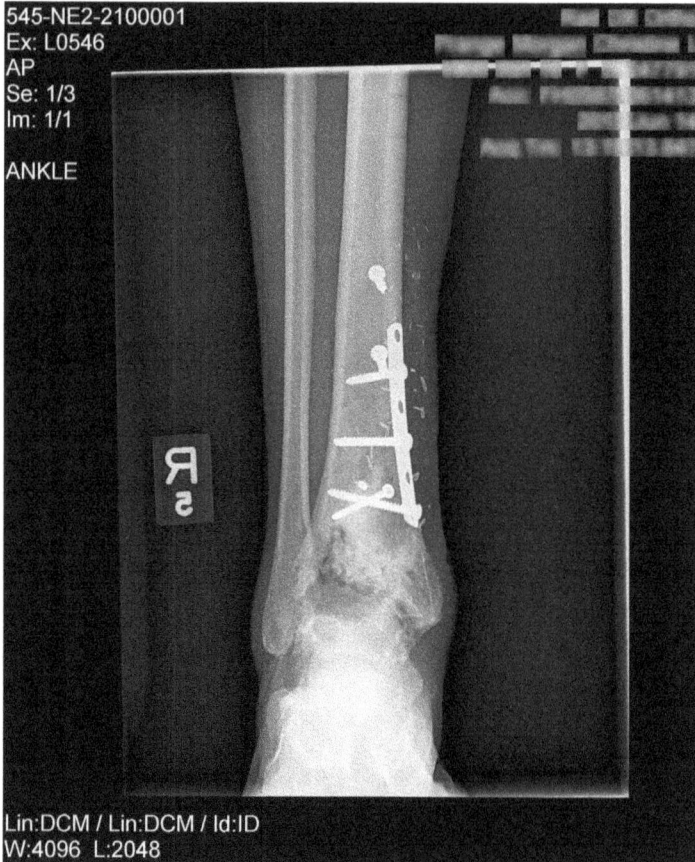

Broken ankle shards, 2011.

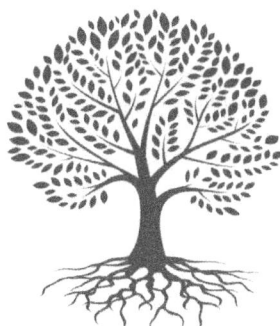

CHAPTER 3

SHAME AND WORTHINESS

HOLDING ON

At 7:30 a.m., a nurse gave me a shot of the anti-anxiety drug Versed to calm my nerves and wheeled me into the operating room to meet the surgeon for reconstructive surgery.

"I'm concerned about your sacrum," the attending said. "It's supposed to be supporting a bundle of nerves that run through the area that controls bowel and bladder function, along with the ability to raise and lower your foot. I won't know until I get in there what the extent of the damage is."

"Bowel and bladder function?" I cried, punching my way through the narcotic-induced calm back into reality and seeing a future where I was wearing adult diapers, using a geriatric walker, living a shadow of the life I once had known. I was thankful to have had a steady stream of medicine pumping into my system by now, with likely an additional bit of Versed to take the edge off my pre-surgery anxiety.

Unable to contain my feelings, my body shuddered involuntarily. A sense of doom clouded my awareness, and I felt overwhelmed by helplessness, terror, and complete despondency.

My mind raced to a former neighbor, Brenda, who had lived with persistent lower back pain and a related condition called "drop foot." Brenda was young, tall, blonde, and attractive, yet tormented—I could see it in her eyes and in the way she hobbled with her old-school silver walker to the bus stop every morning beside her two sandy-blond-haired boys. I felt sympathy for her in her struggle, because it was obvious she was in pain. All I knew was she looked like she was so dang tired and agonized—I knew I was. I couldn't muster up any additional energy to help anyone because I felt I needed my own lifeline thrown, yet nothing was forthcoming. Now, I could really empathize.

My own pent-up frustrations of being a suburban mom seethed just under the surface. I wondered if she felt the same—trying to keep up appearances while concealing the daily anguish behind a forced smile. The perfectly manicured lawns and impeccable homes, sparkling SUVs, and flawless, tailored garden landscapes obscured the contradictory reality of daily meltdowns, agonizing control battles, and my feelings of inadequacy in the realm of motherhood.

In my desert of isolation, I felt immobilized by fear of others' perceptions, real and imagined. The fabled "Momzillas" can be ruthless—and they're real! I felt their judgment lurking around every corner, so I kept my fear and self-doubt hidden behind a crumbling façade of confidence and self-reliance. Maybe my pain wasn't as obvious as Brenda's, but my emotional pain felt just as real.

I had often wondered if I should reach out to my struggling neighbor—I could offer to help her get the kids on the bus, even though their bus stop was a block away in the other direction. I entertained the possibility of connecting with her to ask about her struggles. But the keen, persistent awareness of having my hands *more than full* with Kai corralled any ponderings of supporting my neighbor. How I could I even think about extending myself further? Mornings were hard enough for me to get just my kids ready and out the door on time, with lunches in hand and both shoes on their feet. Through my living room window or from the detached spot of my children's bus stop, I continued to watch Brenda struggle, morning after morning, while I toiled through my own private daily anguish.

One evening when I returned from the grocery store, I noticed a fire truck and slew of squad cars outside Brenda's home. I wondered if she had fallen down the stairs, or if maybe a grandparent was over and had a heart attack. Several days later, while I was waiting with Jade and Kai at our corner bus stop, another mom told me the woman died by suicide.

"I think she shot herself, but I'm not sure."

My heart ached for her, and now for her family. Her sons would grow up without their mom. I felt guilty I hadn't done anything to help her or at least acknowledge to her what I was seeing and feeling when I watched her trek out to the bus stop every morning. If I had struck up a nonchalant conversation about my own feelings of overwhelm and isolation, maybe *she* would've felt understood and less alone. It could have happened naturally because I saw her. I knew the anguish in her eyes because I was steeped in my own suffering—sans the unimaginable physical pain and disability. I was stuck in my own pain and loneliness of mothering a child who could not love me back and sucked every last ounce of energy that I had. I had nothing left to give, yet I still felt ashamed I hadn't reached out to her on one of those mornings.

Brenda's painful life continued to haunt me after her suicide. Did she ever long for her pre-motherhood days? I certainly did. I wondered, *What if Kai hadn't been neglected? What if we got him the day he was born? What if we could've bonded from day one and he could've felt every bit of the love I wanted to give? Could he have loved me back?*

Entrenched in these feelings, my projections of judgment from others haunted me daily. I presume similar feelings haunted Brenda as well. Visions of the terrible things other people might be saying danced in my head.

"Welcome to parenthood."

"Did you think motherhood was supposed to be easy?"

"Maybe you weren't cut out to be a mom and this is payback."

Adding to my feelings of isolation was the painful acknowledgment that no one, other than other parents of children with Reactive Attachment Disorder, would have had any clue what I was experiencing. Unrelenting dread. Sucking the life out of me. Day after hellish day.

Now, laying on the gurney and prepped for surgery, Brenda's story haunted me yet again. I'd been so shackled by my own fear and shame, trying so hard to protect and preserve myself, that I never reached out. I never let on that I was drowning emotionally—physically spent and spiritually wrung out—so much so that I had forgotten who I was. A sense of stark desolation permeated the operating room as the surgeon described my pelvic ring injury and all the potential complications and life-changing symptoms that could happen.

"Will I have chronic pain?" I asked, yearning for a tinge of hope and reassurance that life would return to normal once he put me back together like Humpty Dumpty.

"Probably," he responded way too bluntly, looking at me squarely in the eyes as if I was asking way too many questions he didn't like answering.

My neighbor's desperate fate plagued me. I wondered if I would be in the same position as Brenda—an overwhelmed mom in terrible pain, stuck on the never-ending treadmill of intense parenting responsibilities. I wondered if I would one day want to die, feeling robbed and cheated of a lifetime of relative ease, self-determination, and joy. I welcomed the mask the anesthesiologist was placing over my mouth and nose. Eager to drift off into oblivion, I inhaled deeply.

I recall dreaming that I was mowing the lawn, and when I woke after surgery, I found my hands clasped around the metal bar spanning from hip bone to hip bone. I looked down to see two screws burrowed into each iliac crest, poking out of a holes in my skin which were covered by surgical tape. A dark gray titanium rod bent around my abdomen to keep my pelvis in place, as two additional lag screws had also been driven through my backside, re-connecting my sacrum.

My surgeon said he was pleased at how the surgery went. He believed he was able to subvert the severe neurological damage that could have been the case had he not been able to fit everything back together as well as he did. He also fastened something called an "external fixator" on my lower leg to keep everything stationary for three weeks, until my next reconstruction surgery.

Scott brought Jade and Kai up to my hospital room, and with wide eyes they peppered me with questions about all the metal attachments to my body. Kai was particularly fixated on the foley catheter hanging to the left side of my bed, which was collecting urine as I lay immobile. While we attempted to conceal the tube under the bed sheet, Kai kept poking at the catheter despite our urging him not to.

I felt ashamed of my situation in the first place—needing a tube inserted into my bladder to collect my urine felt gross and disgusting—and I didn't need my child calling further attention to the issue.

A deep anger arose within me, and I barked at Kai, "Get away from there! Stop doing that!"

Embarrassed, feeling vulnerable in my broken condition and mortified at my less-than-stellar ability to parent from my bed, I asked Scott to take the kids home.

The mental gymnastics continued. Why did I persistently feel so responsible for this child who continued to thwart me, even now, in my broken medical condition? I knew he was too young to understand what he was doing, and part of me became angry with Scott for not protecting me from these feelings of continued tension and accountability. Pulling deep from within my inner resolve, I asserted that the hospital environment was not the best place for Kai, as I did not need the additional mental stress of feeling the need to wrangle him in if he pulled at my foley catheter, tried to spin the wheels at the bottom of my portable IV pole, or decided to see what would happen if he forced enough paper towels into my hospital room toilet.

Resentment at my situation slid in like an avalanche, and anger, its loyal counterpart, followed. "What if" thoughts plagued me: *What if I hadn't gotten myself into this predicament? What if I hadn't been so insistent on "saving" this kid, who has become the bane of my existence? What if I had only backed off and taken better care of myself in the first place?*

I toggled between blaming my son for my accident and pardoning him because of his own trauma. Cognitively, I understood the origins and the mechanisms of Kai's pathology. Yet the fallout had a huge effect on our family, and now, the ensuing consequences on me were life-changing and profound. I was pissed. I was sad. I was hopeless and furious and bitter. *Damn this kid.* I felt like the worst mom in the world for having these thoughts, yet this accident was proof of my absolute overwhelm. I welcomed the reprieve from parenting for a while, as these feelings were replaced with ruminations of fear and trepidation about my own wellbeing and future.

I not only felt trapped in a body which was no longer my ally, but also stuck in feelings of pain, of physical and emotional immobility. *Dammit, I can't win.* Bearing the weight of intense guilt and ambivalence about the future, I let go. Who could blame me now for being a bad mom, when, if anything, they might actually feel sorry for me? Maybe folks would even cut me some slack and be forgiving. The real burning question was: *Can I forgive myself for this life-changing mistake?* Could I cut *myself* some slack for not being able to single-handedly fix my son's early trauma, since I now realized that my unwavering resolve to do so had cost me my own wellbeing? Having been unquestionably worn down by parenting, I could now safely abandon the need to be supermom. Nobody would expect it at this juncture, with my broken body. I was relieved and comforted by this awareness.

Hearing about my accident, friends and family members came to the hospital offering all kinds of well wishes. Jade's third grade class made adorable homemade cards, and I had my nurse hang them on the traction pole attached to my bed. Woodside Elementary, Swallow School (where my husband worked), and Willow Springs 4K school offered to help Scott and the kids by delivering cooked meals, and my parents came to assist on the home front while I was in the hospital. People were gracious and helpful—a welcome balm for our family's weariness amidst this emerging reality.

I remained on the trauma floor for ten days, where I received multiple blood transfusions to treat presumed internal bleeding and continued scans and tests. I was also fitted with a TLSO brace for my back. My wonderful nurse Rachel, noticing that Jade had a keen interest in asking all kinds of medical questions, wrote "Mini-nurse Jade" on the white board next to the names of the rest of my care team.

"Would you like to scan your mom's bracelet?" Rachel asked.

"*Can I?* Sure!" Jade quipped, grabbing the scanner and twisting her wrist to line up its red X with the bar code on my bracelet.

"Want to give your mom her medications?" Rachel asked, handing Jade a small plastic cup filled with my morning meds.

Jade's eyebrows raised. Her face lit up as she locked eyes with me, carefully carrying the medication cup and a Styrofoam cupful of water to my bedside. "Here you go, Mom. See? I'm a nurse!"

Seeing my daughter feeling proud and helpful warmed my heart. I wondered if this unique experience would influence her career choices one day. *Would she become a nurse? Would she go into the medical field in the future? Will all these hard, dreadful experiences someday bring forth the fruit of growth—in her? In me? In our family?*

My stay in the hospital followed a routine. Mornings began with my medical team assembled around the bed, talking about my progress and the plan of action for the day and days ahead. Scott secured a cot next to my bed so he could be available for emotional support during my hospital stay. He was not only helpful to me mentally and emotionally, but also practically, as he could ask and answer questions during rounds and take copious notes. Thankfully, through the Family Medical Leave Act, he was able to take 12 weeks of job-protected time off, which was a huge help and so necessary.

Day by day, I inched my way toward recovery. While a huge part of me missed being home with my family, a larger part of me enjoyed the reprieve. I felt as if I had finally gotten a pass, which was more than well-deserved. I so needed a break from the tireless job of parenting Kai, with his continued rejection and thwarting. His tantrums. His passive-aggressive rejection of learning and his vitality-sucking black-hole-like energy. *I had given enough.* I needed all my energy reserves channeled into my *own* hope and healing.

BATTLING INERTIA

Back in May of 2010, when Kai was four, we had been in Virginia meeting with neuropsychologist Dr. Frederickson, who specializes in international adoptions, trauma, and attachment disorders. This doctor's forte was in understanding children with the most troubled orphanage backgrounds. To this day, he is a frequent consultant in cases where kids are deemed "hopeless" or "untreatable."

Most medical providers operate from the assumption that children are raised from birth in conventional families, with at least basic access to medical care, nutrition, and common nurturing—none of which were the case with Kai. None of them knew how to treat a patient that deviated so much from that standard. After exhausting all my local resources in getting help for Kai in his early years, it became clear to me that his issues were not in any way "typical." Through my painstaking, abundant research, it became more and more obvious that we would need to travel to obtain the best possible assessment and plan for our son. My sanity and our future depended on it.

Dr. Fredrickson was a tall, lanky man with a wry smile and a caring yet no-nonsense approach. He was a father of several Romanian adoptees, with an uncanny ability to recognize behavioral patterns and issues typically exhibited by children who'd been kept in horrible orphanage conditions. In Kai, he immediately recognized the signs of profound neglect and early malnutrition.

"He is way too small for a kid his age," Fredrickson said. "His lack of language ability is typical for a child who had very little human contact or may have been kept in a dying room. Have you seen that movie?"

"Yes," both Scott and I replied. We were more than familiar with *The Dying Rooms'* haunting scenes of children left in dark corridors, alone. It felt so affirming to have a professional validate our experience and to know we were finally talking with someone who understood our child and our unique family experience. It felt like a divine reprieve to hand Kai over to a trusted professional for a full eight-hours—someone with a good understanding of Kai's behaviors, with knowledge of and experience with how to deal with them.

Following the full evaluation, comprising two eight-hour days of in-depth neuropsychological/developmental assessments, Scott and I filed into Dr. Fredrickson's humid office. We took our place on the overstuffed gray couches, which were way too comfortable, coaxing me into a relaxed state that contradicted the pounding emotional pressure. I surmised that hundreds of desperate parents had also sat on these couches before us, hoping and pleading for the smallest scraps of optimistic or encouraging information about their children. He sat across from us, smiling, with manilla folder in-hand.

"I like your kid," he started. "He wasn't easy to work with, but none of these kids are. Are you ready?"

I felt a mixture of relief—someone finally "got" our son—and dread—what would Dr. Fredrickson say next?

"It makes me sad to see families like yours that are so broken," he continued. He shared a story of one of his former clients, a mom who died by suicide after years of dealing with a violent son who beat her up regularly, a behavior that is common with children with histories of trauma.

"Sometimes these kids turn violent in their later years. Let's hope that's not going to be the case here. It's clear to me that Kai had very little attention before he came to you. I see kids like him so often, and their brains just don't form well without human contact. His delays are pretty significant, but I have a plan to help him. I'm glad we got him early."

Dr. Fredrickson diagnosed Kai with Pervasive Developmental Disorder, Not Otherwise Specified (PDD-NOS; a condition that he would rather have termed "institutional autism" in our case), in addition to Reactive Attachment Disorder (RAD), ADHD, speech and language and learning disorders, as well as a few other diagnoses that would ultimately be ruled out as time progressed. He encouraged us to consider planning for our son's future in some kind of group home and to squirrel money away in a trust for his ongoing care, projecting that it would be highly unlikely Kai would make enough educational gains to become employable and live independently.

My stomach turned. I longed to crawl back under my rock of denial and persist in fantasizing that we would be the exception to these cases.

I retreated to the office bathroom to let myself fall apart. I felt stymied, paralyzed by dread and worry. I sat cross-legged on the bathroom floor, tears pouring onto my jeans. I grasped the yellow towel hanging off the side of the sink, burying my face in a combination of bitterness and despair. *How would the days ahead pan out? How would I survive? How would we survive?* It seemed unfair that we were stuck in a situation that felt so hopeless.

My problem-solving mind scrambled for coping strategies. *I can handle this*, I reasoned. Yet the landslide of trauma which had permeated our lives had proven far more powerful than I. My meager attempts at shoring up my son's profoundly complex wounds were like trying to erect temporary structures that could withstand the crushing weight of falling earth.

Determined to dig out from under rubble of these earth-shattering psychological diagnoses, I threw cold water on my face. I couldn't let them see how I had begun to crack under the pressure, or how unworthy I felt as a mom saddled with such intense responsibilities. I had to keep myself together and go back in, ready to listen and plan.

I unlocked the bathroom door and returned to the office couch, where I shared my shock and desolation with my husband and Dr. Fredrickson. "I apologize for being gone for so long. It was a lot to take in. I'm feeling a tad overwhelmed right now."

"I know this is hard to hear," Dr. Fredrickson said, "But the good news—and I truly mean this as good news—is that, with these diagnoses I am giving Kai, he will qualify for early intervention services, which will help him make great gains that he otherwise would not have made." We discussed the importance of onboarding a village of supportive professionals to assist us back at home, starting with an intensive treatment program called "Applied Behavioral Analysis" therapy, or ABA, which consisted of 30–40 hours a week of intensive one-on-one treatment. Behavioral intervention programs would turn out to be a huge part of our future; ABA therapy was one of the appointments Kai had to miss on the day I fell from the climbing wall.

I had to relinquish my need for reassurance because no one had a crystal ball. Kai's future was uncertain. But while we had no idea what would be in store for the days and years ahead, we were given permission to ask for help in the form of diagnostic codes. Now we had access to professionals' support outside of our family and tools that would give

Kai the best possible chance of making significant educational, psychological, and developmental gains.

As we returned home from Virginia, I fought hard to resist the apathy and sluggishness that crept in with subtle insidiousness. This would be a marathon, not a sprint—and I always hated long distance.

CLIMBING BACK

Once discharged to inpatient rehab, where I would begin to build strength and navigate my post accident world, I learned I would need to lay flat for a period of three months to allow my pelvic fracture to heal. And my hideous, throbbing right leg would need to remain elevated to keep swelling as manageable as possible. Patience would once again become my reluctant friend.

I hate being patient. I am so much better at swift action, tenacity, and resolve. A problem-solver by nature, now stuck laying in a hospital bed, I continued to ask questions and sought out answers to relieve my anxiety, since I felt so helpless being unable to rush the healing process. This was clearly frustrating for my medical team, who addressed each of my badgering questions and prodding for reassurance with "Everyone is different," or "We will have to see how things go." Obviously, they could not give me the reassurances I wanted. They could not tell me that everything was going to be "normal" again despite my prodding for this answer. I was damn fortunate they liked me.

My rehabilitation stay was punctuated by physical therapy, occupational therapy, dressing/bandage changes, pin-site cleanings, tests, scans, and bloodwork. My schedule was kept tight enough to deplete my energy by the end of the day, leaving me dog-tired and spent by dinner time. My family came to visit every evening, and, despite my physical fatigue, I looked forward to seeing them.

One evening, we watched my fever climb to 103°F. The staff had to ask my family to leave when it became clear I had some type of infection. This would require more antibiotics and another blood transfusion. Perspiration ran down my red-hot face, and my tight-fitting TLSO brace dug painfully into my right side. Every small movement hurt. I felt miserable.

I thought, *Is this bad dream ever going to end?* Wave after wave of disappointment crashed over me. I just wanted to return to normal.

My rehab doctor ordered an X-ray—STAT! This showed a newly fractured rib, something that I was informed would have to heal on its own. The nurses administered more pain medicine. I ended up with a bad case of hives, likely an allergic reaction to my bleached sheets or one of the medications, and I struggled to fight the urge to scratch my skin until it bled.

"Don't scratch," they said.

Ugh! I was so damned uncomfortable. This was made worse by the fact that my hair had only been washed once in the last two weeks. The smell of dead skin, greasy hair, and dried blood permeated my room. I felt disgusting.

Being a patient can feel dehumanizing. Medical staff are overworked and pressed for time. Sometimes they don't have time to answer questions. The can be abrupt and cold. Outside clothes are taken away and replaced with a starchy pastel hospital gown. Any identity is stripped away and replaced by the malady which now defines you: I was a "trauma patient."

I fought hard to focus on the pride of survivorship. I was determined to come out still kicking ass, despite the overwhelming inertia which threatened to pull me under more and more swiftly with each new setback.

Being a competitive athlete had given me a bit of an advantage in life: a stubborn determination to turn things around and to come out on top. Yet even a determined athlete has her tipping point. With each unrelenting wave, each new inevitable obstacle, I would wonder how much more erosion my spirit could handle before crumbling entirely.

Summoning the inner resolve to keep going after repeated setbacks will wear away at any living entity, beginning at the cellular level. I began to see this physiological response in my own body, at the end of my second week of hospitalization, when the phlebotomist came in for routine bloodwork.

The insides of my arms and the tops of my hands began to look as if I had been badly beaten, with various stages of black and blue marks and with yellow pock marks running up and down my arms as if I was a heavy IV drug user. My veins quivered and rolled from side to side each time the needle approached my tender skin for another blood draw, as if they had learned through experience that yet another bodily insult approached.

"I swear that people's veins develop minds of their own," one phlebotomist said, as I watched her attempt to find a good vein to stick. "It's as if they see me coming, and they get scared."

"Wow," I replied. "You see this a lot? Veins jumping around to avoid the needle?"

"If patients have been here for a while, it's like something in people's blood or their veins learns to say, 'Yikes! Here she comes again!'" she added. "I always feel bad when I go into patient rooms. They never want to see me—their veins scream, 'Not her again!'"

My mind darted to my son. Analogous to my quivering veins, I wondered if Kai's psyche had developed a visceral aversion to maternal love and affection, a learned behavior since his earliest moments were also laden with psychic insult in the form of parental abandonment, orphanage trauma, and institutional neglect. His resistance to me certainly appeared just as instinctive and involuntary as my quivering veins. This was a deeply profound revelation, one I would keep in mind in the years to come.

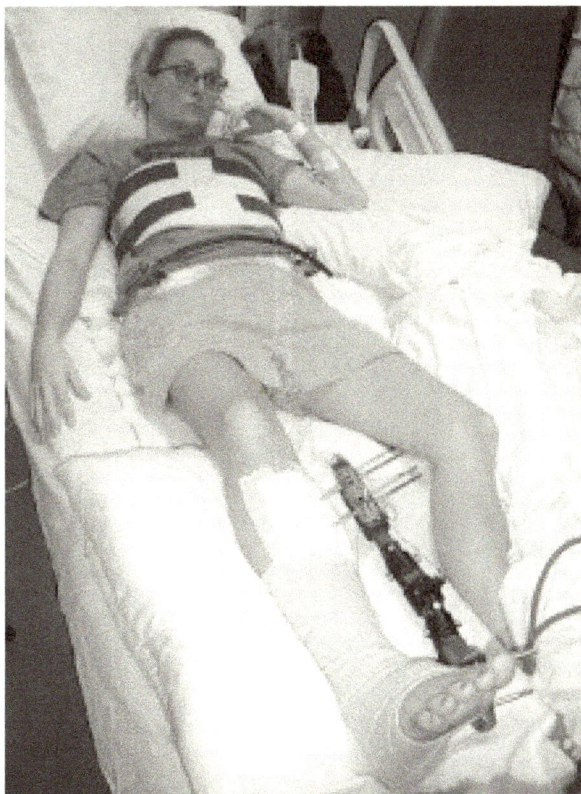

Post–accident, December, 2011.

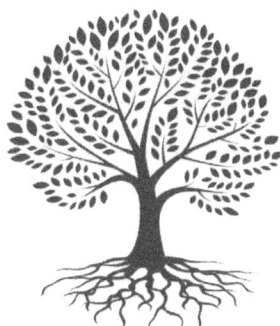

CHAPTER 4

PAIN AND PERSISTENCE

PAIN AND BEING HEARD

The evening of my first ankle reconstruction surgery, I was in profound, excruciating pain. I had returned to my hospital room after the morning's anesthesia wore off, and a hot, achy, searing pain rushed into my lower right leg. I pushed the red call button to request that a nurse come to my room. Ten minutes passed until she came to my bedside. Sweat had begun to roll down my brow.

"I'm sorry I couldn't get here earlier. I was with another patient," she said. "How are you? How is your pain?"

"Ugh. It's really bad," I replied. "I don't think I can take it much longer. Can you give me something?"

"What would you rate your pain on a scale of one to ten?"

I hated the stupid, subjective pain scale. I could not give my pain a "10" because that was supposed to mean "I'm about to pass out." All my life I had endured a very high pain tolerance, but now I felt like my ankle was going to explode. I gave my pain an "8." Scott sat to the left of my bed while I squeezed his hand, writhing and moaning.

"I've never seen Chris like this," he shared with my nurse. "The pain has got to be really bad for her to be whimpering like this."

"Let me put in a call to your doctor to get an order to increase your pain meds," she replied.

Can't she just give me something right now? I wondered. I wanted to crawl out of my skin. Nothing would console me. I couldn't focus on anything or engage in conversation with Scott as he tried to comfort me. All I could do was continue to writhe and moan.

At least an hour had passed and now my pain level was at a "9." It was around 1:30 a.m. and it felt like I'd been waiting an eternity. I pressed my call light again. I felt like I was going to pass out from the unrelenting agony. I wanted to die. The nurse came back into my room.

"I paged the resident on call, and I'm still waiting for his response. I'm sorry. I know you're in pain and it's hard to hang in there."

At this point I was in so much pain that I had no filter. I couldn't believe that they had let me go this long. I now knew why people with prolonged untreated chronic pain took their lives. I was furious.

"You're sorry? No, I'm sorry!" I yelled. "You get on the phone with my doctor now! I don't care what it takes! I'm in fucking pain! *Don't you CARE?*"

Scott rubbed my arm. I could tell he was embarrassed. I had probably woken up the entire hospital ward.

"Yeah, this isn't Chris," he said. "She isn't usually like this. Please. Get her doctor on the line now."

Within about 15 minutes, the resident on call showed up at my bedside. He was a tall, young guy with sandy blond hair, which sported an obvious bedhead. He walked to the end of my bed and put his fingers under my cast, above my toes. "Do you feel that?"

"No." I responded, still writhing in agony.

He proceeded to take out long specialized scissors and cut down the middle of my cast. I began to feel some relief and realized that my leg had been swelling under the cast with nowhere to expand. He pried the right side of the cast out a bit and touched my skin with the cool stainless steel of the scissors.

"Do you feel that?"

"Yes, I can feel that."

"That's good," he reassured me. "I wanted to rule out something called 'compartment syndrome,' which can be life-threatening. I think you are just swelling a lot and I needed to relieve the pressure by loosening the cast." He ordered an increase in my pain medication, which provided a welcome relief.

"Thank you for getting here," I said to him. "I'm sorry, I probably got you out of bed."

He apologized for not getting to me earlier, mumbling something about sleeping heavily and not hearing the pager right away. I felt bad for yelling at my nurse, yet I couldn't help myself. I was in so much pain—it had to go somewhere.

Scott and I slept well as my pain became better controlled and the pressure in my leg was alleviated as the swelling was given some space to expand. I had never experienced that kind of agony before, and I never wanted to experience it again.

Years later, when I began working as a hospital chaplain, when I'd find myself at the bedside of patients in intense pain, I would advocate for them. I understand well the tough demands in medicine and busyness required to meet them. I also know that pain ain't no joke. Pain can turn us into monsters if it is ignored or brushed under the rug. Like the Incredible Hulk, its power has the ability to unearth a quaking, momentous force that causes us to act crazy and irrational. All pain— physical, spiritual, and emotional—sucks. It causes us to do things that we later regret. All organisms in pain seek comfort and release from its obstinate grasp.

HOME

I was discharged from the hospital on December 24, 2011. It was a brisk, cold winter day. Scott pulled his Honda Accord up to the hospital entrance, where I sat waiting in a wheelchair. I felt comforted and happy to be going home. The cold air felt refreshing as Scott and the staff gingerly helped to slide me into the back seat and covered me with a light blue fleece blanket, lying on my back with my foot elevated.

I was relieved I had bought everyone's Christmas gifts ahead of time, including sleds for the kids, new fleece pajamas, and child-sized snow shovels that would fortuitously come in very handy this year. I was also thankful we had decided to put up and trim the tree the day after Thanksgiving—just four days before my accident.

A homecare medical agency had set up a hospital bed in the corner of the living room, with the Christmas tree at the opposing corner, just at the foot of my bed.

"Mom, you might get to see Santa!" Jade exclaimed. I laughed at this suggestion, knowing I'd probably be way too crashed out to even care.

We set up a table next to the bed with my medications and a journal to record each time I took them. A commode and a rose-colored bedpan sat in front of the table. I felt a twinge of embarrassment, having all these necessities out in the main room of our house for all to see. My kids kept me focused on lighter things, like presents, treats, and Santa. I was grateful for family and friends who came to lift our spirits and bring some welcome levity. We tried as hard as we could to make the winter holidays seem fun and exciting for the kids, even though our lives had been turned upside down. The "most wonderful time of the year" didn't feel very wonderful, but we did our best to make it so for the kids.

As we entered the new year, I was both thankful that this ordeal was happening during the most miserable time of the year and worried about what the ensuing months would bring. It started to become more and more obvious to me that my body was not going to just bounce back. Feelings of panic and isolation started to set in. *What if I never get back to normal? What if I am stuck here, in this painful body, in my private hell of parenting a child who cannot love me back? What if there is absolutely no winning in this game—no silver lining? Can I go on in this life if all I continue to experience is more pain and heartbreak? More suffering?*

Thinking about the days, weeks and years ahead, I could not grasp what a life well-lived would now look like. I secretly hoped I would waste away, or at least, fall asleep peacefully and not wake up. Maybe I would be lucky and get cancer from all the scans and X-rays, ushering me swiftly out. My mind was restless, thinking of ways to escape this pitiful, torturous life I now inhabited—bereft of pleasure and overshadowed by anguish, with the certainty of more suffering now on the immediate horizon.

The person I had been was now lost forever. My sunny character and everything about the person I knew myself to be had been lost in the shadow of my former pre-accident self. A strong sense of shame and worthlessness began sneaking in, and I deemed that I would become a wretched, sullen person—a drain on society and a solemn burden to my family. I thought about my neighbor who had taken her life. My thoughts turned dark and ugly. *There may no longer be a place for me here,* I thought.

Having a background in clinical mental health, I knew that if I shared these feelings with anyone in the field they'd think I was suicidal. Comments that seem hopeless and dark are guaranteed to prompt the question of suicidality, and I certainly didn't want folks worrying about me. Even though I skirted those edges, my husband continued to remind me to take things one day, or even *one step*, at a time.

Scott would encourage me: "Chris, just take the damned pain meds. I don't like seeing you in so much pain. That is what they're for."

I was reluctant to keep taking opiate pain medication for fear of becoming addicted, having heard the stories and knowing of folks who didn't know when to stop and later finding themselves detoxing at drug treatment facilities.

"Ugh. I don't *want* to take them! But the pain is so bad when I don't take 'em though, or if I get behind."

Sighing, with tears welling up in my eyes, the words fell out of my mouth: "If this is how life is going to be—if I have to live with this kind of pain—I don't know if I want to be here anymore. I can't live like this. I just can't."

"Chris, I know it's hard. Don't let your mind go there," Scott said. "We'll get through this. I need you. The kids need you."

The kids need you. Hrumph, I thought. My daughter was a ray of sunshine who could brighten my world. My son, however, brought me more pain and heartbreak with each mounting day. I couldn't even think about parenting him in the days ahead, since I still needed all my energy for my own healing.

"You'll have to pick up the slack with Kai, Scott." I said. "*I just can't.*"

"Of course I will," Scott assured me, noting that all the work I had put into Kai's early interventions had now taken hold, and Kai was well taken care of with 30 hours a week of in-home therapies.

Scott proceeded to remind me that my body had been injured in ways that were going to take time to heal. We talked about the fact that there would be bad days and good days, and Scott assured me that my pain wouldn't last forever. But I wasn't so sure. All I knew was that I now felt extremely alone in my pain, and that there was no end in the foreseeable future. The thought of continuing to live in this life felt like looking down an empty, dank, cavernous tunnel without an exit. My world had once been a sunny, fertile mountaintop of boundless opportunity where I could harness the beauty and adventure I knew waited around every corner. Now, I was stuck, feeling hopeless and utterly resentful.

Why had I brought this child into our lives who caused me to be so keyed up and unearthed a side of me that I absolutely could not stand?

How could I have been so damned insistent that we save this child from the other side of the world, only to have this shit happen? I felt like I would be living in anguish and despair forever. I now hated myself for my need to fix and save the world, because I could not save myself.

I was stuck. I was in pain. I hated what my life had become.

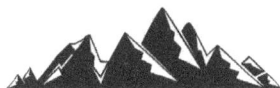

Back home, I didn't have the distraction of medical tests, hospital rounds, or conversations with medical folks who "got it" to hold my attention. Drenched in resentment and looking ahead at a hard life trajectory, I allowed myself to sprawl out on the living room floor and lose it, picking at the gray flecks in the carpet as tears slowly ran down my face. Lying in a lump on the floor, it occurred to me that this was the same carpeted floor my son oozed upon in his earliest days with us, transfixed by the wheels of his matchbox cars and zoning out in a little world of his own. Massaging my fingers through the texture of the rug, I wondered if Kai's tears and thoughts of despair had trickled into these same fibers in his hardest days. Now the carpet held a double dose of dread.

In the ongoing tug-of-war in my thinking, I realized that this mandatory stillness meant I was forced to behold the beautiful in the littlest details, from a wheelchair in my kitchen with an elevated, casted foot. It was this mindfulness that got me through. By managing to bring my attention to life's smallest features—the softness of my cat's plush fur, the sick-humored banter between my caring husband and parents, the scent of my kids' freshly shampooed hair just after bath time—I was able to cope with the arduousness of the moments which came and went each day. In time, my darkened thoughts began to brighten, despite the mounting daily challenges.

Feeling like the "eternal patient," my life felt centered around waiting for medical appointments, medications, and news about my shattered ankle, which would require more surgeries. I started to look into ways I could weave more of these smallish bits of gratitude into my life by simply noticing more, because my life had slowed down enough to perceive the world around me with greater intensity. Pain continued and, at times, intensified. Yet joy was also magnified. Milkshakes tasted like heaven and the birds at the feeder became my peeping little friends, ready to greet me from the window every sunny April morning. My life's rhythms mirrored the earth's rhythms—the weeping of the rain, followed by the promise of sunshine and the kiss of the gentle spring breezes. *Why*, I wondered, *should my life look any different?*

In the days that followed, I made a distinct effort to pay attention to all the things I *could* find pleasure in. We termed our fluffy tabby cat, Oscar, "the counselor cat," as he had an uncanny intuition for when I was having a rough day. Peering at me from across the room with his slow-blinking, little eyes, he just knew when I needed a snuggle. I welcomed him into my lap with open arms, a scratch under the chin, and another exhale in gratitude, ushered in by his gentle vibrating purr.

Oscar had broken his little paw as a kitten when the kitchen screen door slammed shut as my dad was leaving the room one day. Fortunately, it did not require surgery, but because he had broken it on the growth plate, we were informed that it could cause Oscar problems with arthritis as he became older. The little rascal chewed through two casts before we realized they were causing him too much distress and removed them. Eventually, the bone healed on its own.

I continued to wonder if this experience of Oscar's rendered him more compassionate and sensitive, as shown by his frequent locked-on gaze and slow, blinking kitty kisses. His gentle purr and loving expression helped me feel connected and understood—as if he knew at a deep level what I was feeling. Stroking his soft and fuzzy, warm striped coat, Oscar helped me to know that life was still okay, if only for a moment.

The hospital bed in our living room (with me in it) invited pets and kids to gently come aboard to get in their snuggle time. One chilly afternoon, I invited Jade and Kai to join me under the blankets in their fleece-lined pajamas while I read them the story *Go, Dog. Go!*. Kai giggled in excitement—this felt like a first, as usually he had no interest in snuggling.

"Go dog, go!" he pointed to the hound in the car.

"Vroom vroom!" I smiled, not knowing how long this feeling would last.

In the warm glow of the lamplight, we all became drowsy and dozed off before I reached the middle of the book. Peacefully, I awakened to see my two little ones nestled tightly under each arm, both curled up with rosy cheeks and exuding unencumbered serenity. I wondered if they needed this experience to feel confident and secure again—to know that Mommy was going to get better, and was still here to provide warmth and comfort in the aftermath of all the upheaval.

I wanted to capture this moment in time—their warm little bodies, trusting and vulnerable, snugly radiating that all was right in the world for the moment. Shoring up my broken, pieced-together, hardware-laden body were these two pudgy little bookends.

Looking down at my snoring son, a profound sense of gratitude blanketed the moment with a deep, abiding awareness that for now, things were okay. Kai had trusted me enough to fall asleep with his nose in my armpit. He trusted me enough to be vulnerable, praise God. I didn't know about tomorrow or what the future would bring our way, and in that instant, I didn't care.

SETBACKS

It's hard to get used to having setbacks, but somehow I did, and our family managed to hang on in the turbulent wake of each one. It took some time and persistence to develop a setback hardiness, but humor and determination helped.

Shortly after returning home from my first hospitalization, I noticed an angry redness developing on my skin at the pin sites attaching my external fixator to the front of my hips. This angry redness was accompanied by an oozing yellow drainage, which had the concerning connotation of infection. My homecare nurse put in a phone call to my orthopedic surgeon's office stat, landing us an emergency appointment late that Tuesday evening, sandwiched between resident interviews.

In his office, I was greeted by a team of eager residents and medical students along with my orthopedic doctor and the tech, all keen to get a look at this festering pin site infection.

"Her body's not liking it in there. It's gotta come out," my orthopod uttered with the same blunt matter-of-factness he always did.

"What? Here? Now?" I retorted.

"We don't want the infection to spread, and if we wait until an OR spot opens, we're taking that risk. It won't take long..."

I gasped in fear and complete disbelief that I would once again experience another painful, excruciating medical procedure while awake. I would be slightly sedated, but not unconscious. It felt like an intimate bodily assault, and I was powerless to do anything about it other than suck it up, grit my teeth, and bear the burden. I knew I had handled tough situations before, like when my femur was drilled through in the emergency room. I never realized that my body would continue to feel like a struggling, haphazard construction site, and me, the frustrated un-consulted subcontractor.

Man, this is my BODY, I thought. How odd to be watching this all happen to myself, as if my body was just some kind of hunk of meat. Part of me thought watching this happen was fascinating, because it was a new and deeper slice of life than I had ever imagined. Yet mostly, it felt horrifyingly disturbing and awful. A sense of numbness and subjection came over me as I readied myself for what came next.

Gary, the technician, returned with a socket wrench in hand, still surrounded by the new medical residents clamoring to get in on the action and see his workmanship firsthand. I felt oddly like the Tuesday evening entertainment, but that didn't bother me all that much; I was way too nervous and preoccupied.

"Wow," Scott uttered in surprise. "That's a Sears Craftsman you're using? *Really?*"

Gary held up the socket wrench and cocked his head to the side, mumbling something about the operation not being all that complicated.

"Repairing bodies really is so much like the craft of carpentry," Gary joked. "That's kind of what orthopedics is when it comes down to it."

I looked at Scott and asked if I could squeeze his hand while Gary bore down with his wrench on the four lag screws embedded in each of my iliac crests. I didn't want to watch, and neither did Scott. We held each other's gaze and squeezed hard, both wincing for what seemed like longer than I had anticipated. I felt a deep, creaking ache spread through my hips as a tear snuck out of the corner of my eye and ran down my cheek.

"I guess now I know what a decking board feels like," I jested, feeling the rotating screws screeching out one at a time. Despite the pain medication I had been on at the time, it hurt. A lot. The pain was searing and hot. I'm a pretty tough cookie, but *still...* I was wrung out and just done feeling like I was an unwitting victim of a horrible physical assault. Obviously, I knew I had no choice—this was all fallout from my body's trauma. When it was over, Scott kissed my forehead and put his arm around my shoulder, pulling me close.

"Yeah," he said. "That was pretty intense." I thanked him for holding my hand and not passing out this time around.

Wheeling me back to the car, Scott chuckled a sigh of relief and mumbled something about the truth behind the vows "for better or worse." Feeling a bit shaky and overwhelmed, I was thankful to have him by my side.

For three months, I spent most of my days lying flat, with my pounding right leg elevated on three pillows. A dingy gray commode sat beside my bed, still situated in the corner of the living room.

"It's a bird. It's a plane. It's *commode-man!*" I joked, feeling embarrassed and horrified that Scott needed to empty it after each use. Scott would roll his eyes and chuckle as he grabbed the silver handle of the commode pail with an outstretched arm and carried it into the bathroom for disposal.

With the right footrest elevated, I used a wheelchair to get into the kitchen and to appointments. Scott drove me to every appointments while I reclined in the back seat with my right leg propped up on a pillow. I had never felt like a "high maintenance" person before this, and I didn't like it. I felt guilty for needing so much help, and I apologized over and over.

"Sorry, Scott. I feel so bad—this is all so disgusting."

My homecare nurse continued to come to our house daily to check my vitals, change my bandages, and bring a bit of education and levity. She would notice and document each small detail or concern. Weeks were punctuated by checkup visits to my orthopod's office, always laden with anticipatory dread. Like going into battle, I started to gear up emotionally for the setbacks I now expected—it seemed inevitable that they would come after every welcomed reprieve. I began to wonder *why*. What was the universe trying to teach me? Why had I been forced to continue enduring such unrelenting pain—in so many aspects? When would I get my life back? *Would I ever find relief?*

Looking for a way to process what I was going through, I began to consider that a seed will not sprout until it is cracked open. The seed is not asked if it is okay with this predicament. It is just beckoned by the rain and sun's persistence. I was no different. I could either choose to grow through being cracked open, again and again, or wither away, allowing pain, sorrow, and bitter resentment to rot the husk containing the hardiness at my core. With each unrelenting setback, I made the choice to tend to my inner resilience, to find ways to nourish this tenderly sprouting seedling of resolute growth.

As I continued to recover and explore the various new insights and limitations in my body, the power of nature was an ever-abiding reminder that restoration and rebuilding takes time. We can't force it. *I* couldn't force it—neither in my own body nor in my son's psyche. Pain and healing are inseparable forces coexisting in dynamic tension with one another, always summoned by transcendence and growth—aching to be *better*, somehow. While I could certainly work with the process by eating well, going to physical therapy, and trying to stay in a good headspace, my body's return to health would continue to be a dance with the universe, independent of my wants. My son's journey toward emotional health, connection, and maturity took its course alongside my process. The north star of healing and becoming whole again awaited, just outside of our grasp.

In order to stay in a good headspace, I needed four things: something to look forward to (an experience), something to work toward (a goal), people around me whom I cared about (companionship), and the healing power of the outdoors (nature). Even with an uncertain future, a non-healing ankle, and persistent lower back pain, I knew for sure that I could find something pleasant to focus on to get through each day.

In April, when I could finally hobble about on crutches, I slowly made my way over the patchy grass and the damp woodchips to the cedar playset in the corner of the yard where both the kids had assembled a pretend "operating room" on the top of the green slide tower. Jade's stuffed dog, Pink Puppy, and tiger, Cleo, were the subjects. Both Kai and Jade donned their blue latex gloves and took the patients' vitals.

"Wook, Mom," Kai said. "Cweo is sick."

"And I think Pink Puppy has an infection. He needs IV antibiotics," Jade piped in, taking off her stethoscope, having finished pretending to find Cleo's pulse.

"Oh no! I hope they're both okay!" I laughed, smiling widely as the kids kept going with their imaginary clinic.

I noticed both stuffed animals had wrist bands with their names on them. The kids took turns scanning their bands and giving out medications. My kids knew their medical shtick well, and it made my heart happy to watch them.

As time went on, Jade continued to have an interest in healthcare, with excellent grades and ambition to support her goals. Kai would began turning his imagination play toward pretend cooking, acquiring an interest in making "real food" and later taking a culinary arts class. His household chore of clearing the dinner table and loading the dishwasher came in handy as he developed quite the knack for stacking dishes and multitasking. His surplus of energy was definitely helpful on the days I didn't have an extra ounce to spare.

I began to appreciate that, despite my incapacity and the hardships our family had encountered, my little ruffians would find their creative spaces in the universe. In spite of our struggles and pain, we didn't just endure. We persisted in our challenges and grew. And I was happy.

THE SUMMIT OF HOPE

Laying in that hospital bed in my living room in the early days of 2012, I so intensely wanted to heal. I read books on visualization, ate well, and tried to exude enough positive thoughts to part the seas, yet I could not will my ankle to heal. Pain remained. Surgeries had continued into January, where I'd spent two more weeks in the hospital. Then at a follow-up visit in March, one of my doctors referred to my situation as "limb salvage." That caught my attention. *Salvage?* I wondered. Like, as in salvage yard for old, broken automobiles? The thought was poignant and disheartening.

Kai's development continued to lag, and his ability to connect was—despite my best efforts—still a challenge at times. Often snapping at or avoidant of Scott and the kids, I was an irritable and cranky hot mess with a very short fuse, made worse by unresolved pain as the days wore on. I began to feel useless, ineffective, and powerless, and I longed for something to propel me out of my deep dark funk.

As the reality of our circumstances continued to unfold, I started searching for ways we could continue to enjoy being family together with activities which were active and non-sedentary. I knew that I would lose my mind if we didn't find a way to get out of the house and travel somewhere beautiful together where I could get moving and find my bearings in nature. I so longed for beauty and fresh air to reinvigorate the stagnant world we had begun to inhabit in our house of ongoing convalescence.

Sometime in mid-March, sandwiched in between the blur of ongoing surgeries and medical appointments, I began scouring the internet for inspirational stories of other trauma survivors. I wanted to know how they had risen from the ashes and how they had found the inner strength to persist despite continued challenges and setbacks. Between recovering from injury and parenting, I felt as if my resiliency-response system was stuck in overdrive. I craved the balm of others' good energy to validate the struggle I was experiencing day after day. I knew I needed some kind of push from outside myself to gain the strength and momentum to keep going. I needed to find new ways to embrace joy and adventure as a person with a disability while also parenting a child with a unique type of developmental disability. This life of ours was indeed different from the norm, and it required a new and creative game plan.

In my detailed quest for connection, I came upon a gem of an organization called No Barriers, based out of Fort Collins, Colorado. No Barriers' motto, "What's within you is stronger than what's in your way," resonated with me immediately. I understood well the insidious, quicksand-like inertia that could creep in through daily trials of persistent pain and barriers to living fully. I felt the lure of self-pity and depression lurking around in my life's shallow corners and I fought fiercely against their strong forces. It became increasingly evident that these new challenges would be here for the long haul, and I wanted to embrace an empowering mindset which could get us through.

For the first time since my climbing fall, I felt my adventurous spirit and lust for life returning. This was an important breakthrough in healing emotionally, because it re-grounded me back within myself after I felt I had lost so much of who I was. The 2012 No Barriers Summit in Telluride, Colorado, would be just the thing to ignite that quest for adventure and camaraderie with like-minded folks. Preparing for a drive through the mountains to get to an event promising hope flooded me with a new spiritual invigoration, which spilled over into the family. The mom my family knew was finally starting to come back, and we were excited for our adventure.

The Summit is an activity-based event focused on creating community, challenging perceived barriers, and re-defining what is possible for folks with challenging life circumstances and their families. Hearing the inspirational stories from all kinds of people who faced incredible adversity—limb loss, blindness, paralysis and other hardships—I gained a new appreciation for the concept of strength. My perception had typically focused on physical strength and tenacity—winning medals, working long hours, or bragging about impressive physical feats. I was starting to see and feel something altogether different: an inner strength which emerged from deep within, beckoned into the light where the mental head game of healing can't be separated from the emotional or the physical, and the support of others is crucial.

Eight months after my accident, still on crutches and lugging a heavy ankle boot, I found ways to hike through the mountains in a community of others who took things more slowly. I was able to rock climb on top-rope (with a few adaptations and without using my bad ankle) alongside folks with more difficult circumstances—among them, a bilateral above-knee amputee, an arm amputee, and a traumatic brain injury survivor.

I watched in amazement as Scott and Jade chatted intimately with people about their stories of resilience and survival while Kai listened, occasionally asking, appropriately, "What's that?" or "What happened?" It occurred to me that my kids were absorbing the priceless stories of real-life heroes in real time. While Kai was a bit more limited in his understanding, Jade was intrigued by the stories she heard. At the end of the four-day event, Jade commented, "I don't think of these people as being different for having disabilities. They just seem 'normal.'" I loved that this rich, experiential learning opportunity took my children out of the ordinary and expanded their minds and worlds. They were immersed in a life-changing experience which impacted not only them, but also their mom.

Sitting at dinner in the Summit's large white tent with my family, I looked briefly to my left to see a group of three young female amputees running with curved carbon-fiber running blades. I began to feel a twinge of jealousy as I noted their lighthearted nature and ease as they bounced by me with these sparkly carbon-fiber feet. *Why are they so carefree and happy? They are missing their feet and legs, and I'm not!* In contrast, I was hauling around a puffy, red, swollen ankle, cobbled-together and contained in a heavy black boot. I still used crutches to avoid bearing weight on my ankle eight long months after my accident, and an additional bone graft surgery was on the horizon. Every time I sat down, I needed to elevate my foot to keep it from pounding, and I kept a small container of pain medication in my pocket for the inevitable pain surge. The prospect of amputation—a reality I never thought I'd come to embrace—was beginning to look more appealing than my current circumstances. I began asking questions of the amputees I met during the event.

"What happened that you lost your leg?"

"How long did it take for you to heal?"

"What is it like to put on a prosthetic leg every morning?"

"Do you ever have fitting problems? How do you deal with that?"

"Can you drive?" (I was very interested to know the answer to that one. As long as my right foot was in the boot, I couldn't. And that sucked.)

I approached several different prosthetic providers set up at the vendor tents and asked questions about their experiences with people like me—folks enduring multiple surgeries to salvage their limbs, yearning for a better quality of life. I shared the heartache I experienced, watching my husband and children run around, being active without me, and the pity-party I often threw for myself during these times. With the information I was gathering here, it became increasingly apparent that I could regain my quality of life if I could wrap my head around living life as an amputee. Of course, that would mean chopping my leg off somewhere below the knee, and I was quite attached to my foot, literally.

I dug deep to fortify my inner badass and began to feel lighthearted again. Happiness was once more within reach. My sense of adventure was still intact. My willingness to ask hard questions and confront potential loss was still there. I saw and met firsthand examples of folks living a life I could have, if only I could rid myself of the painful ball-and-chain that was my ankle. While I wasn't quite ready for that, I knew it was always an option. I had a potential "out." I wouldn't be stuck forever.

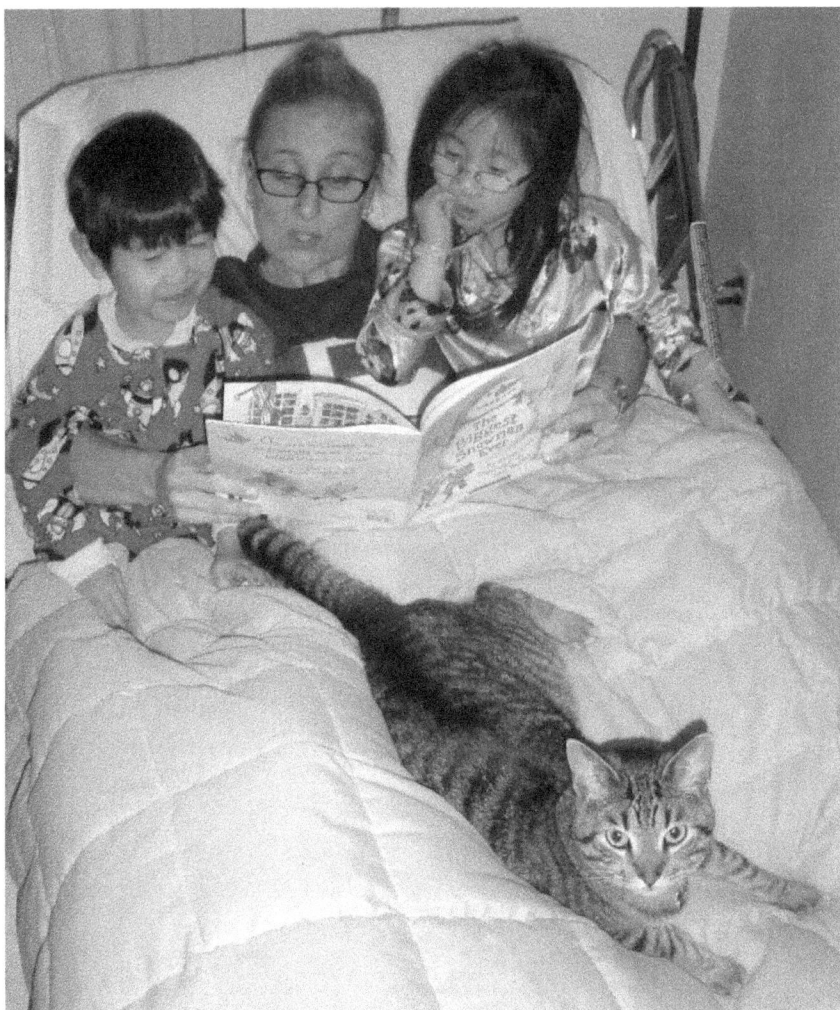

Reading time with my hoodlums, 2011.

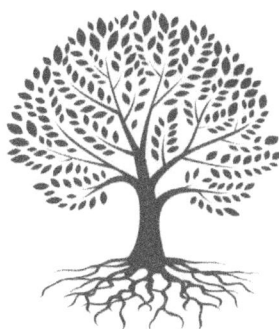

CHAPTER 5

LOSS AND INTEGRITY

STICKY FINGERS

One bright spring morning in 2013, when Kai was seven and Jade was nine, I discovered a surprise after the kids left for school. I went upstairs with the routine intention of getting Kai's laundry, only to notice the nozzle of a brown bottle poking out from under the dangling navy denim sheet of his bed. I was flabbergasted to find an industrial-size bottle of Hershey's Chocolate Syrup! The bottle was empty, of course—I knew he had drunk it all. The huge bottle was not something that was ever in our fridge, and I wondered where he heisted it from.

It is common for kids with histories of trauma to have issues with hoarding, stealing, and food, and our son was no exception. There were the aforementioned calls from school that Kai had scoured other children's school lockers for treats and devoured their bag lunches. If we didn't keep an eye on him, he'd down an entire jar of cookies. He stole books and school supplies from his teachers and other students, and he was always the kid to drag his heels (a form of control) while the rest of the class waited to go to lunch. It was frustrating for us and the school staff, who were helpful, understanding, and supportive but also had limits to *their* patience. Early neglect, malnutrition, and trauma will create these types of behaviors, and they are hard to squelch.

I placed the large empty bottle of Hershey Syrup in the middle of the kitchen table. It was prominent enough that Kai could not miss it when he walked in the door after school. It would stay there until Scott also got home from work so we could have a little chat about this sneaky little heist.

At 3:30 that afternoon, Jade walked in the door behind Kai and immediately noticed the large bottle on the table. She pointed to it and asked, "What's that for?"

"Well, I found this under Kai's bed this morning. Isn't that silly? Why would Kai have a huge bottle of Hershey's syrup in his bedroom, and where did he get it?"

Kai looked at me like a deer in the headlights. He was busted and he knew it.

"Kai, where did you get this?" I asked.

"I dunno," Kai replied. This was his typical response whenever he would get caught for doing something sneaky or out of line.

"I think he stole it from the refrigerator at the climbing gym," Jade chirped. "I know they have those big bottles of syrup for birthday parties."

"Oh, I see." I looked squarely at Kai. It was becoming apparent just how messed up our family was after my accident. "So you stole the bottle, drank the whole thing, and then hid it under your bed?"

Around this time, Scott had come home and seemed curious as to why I was holding a huge bottle of chocolate syrup. I caught him up quickly, and he smacked the palm of his hand on his forehead, shaking his head back and forth.

"You what?" he asked, looking at Kai, knowing that he would not get an answer.

Scott and I peered at each other and simultaneously agreed that Kai would need to take the bottle back to the gym and fess up. He would need to apologize to the staff for stealing, replace the full bottle with his own allowance money, and he would receive some kind of task for retribution. We wanted him to take responsibility for his behavior, even though we figured the staff would probably just laugh and let Kai off the hook.

Scott drove Kai to the gym the following day, with a full replacement bottle of Hershey's Syrup in hand. Zach, one of the gym managers, met them at the desk, and Kai was forced to give an apology.

"I'm sorry." Kai uttered, looking down at the ground.

"Look at Zach, Kai," Scott encouraged.

"Okay. *Sawree.*" Kai continued. "I won't do it again." At the age of eight, Kai was now beginning to understand that there were consequences for his behaviors and people who cared enough about him to hold him accountable to change.

"I hope he didn't get sick," Zach said. Zach is a really nice, friendly guy, inclined to let these kinds of things slide. Scott insisted that Kai make an apology and hand over both the new bottle of syrup and an "I'm sorry" letter for the rest of the management to read. Of course, this was seen as somewhat comical by the staff, as they'd also caught our son stealing Clif Bars and bags of M&Ms from the retail shelf in the past. They knew Kai and our family well enough to know that we had our hands full. We were grateful for their understanding and were completely onboard when Scott insisted that (after all of Kai's shenanigans) Kai clean the insides of all the lockers with soap and a damp sponge as payback.

While annoying and frustrating, these behaviors lessened dramatically over the years but never completely went away. Kai's instinct to hoard stuff and squirrel away food and belongings stems from a background of deep, profound loss. Loss of trust. Loss of hope. Loss of confidence that he would be okay—because, at the time these patterns were formed, he wasn't. The pathways in Kai's brain became wired for survival when they should have been forming bonds with people who cared about and nurtured him. Most children grow up feeling safe. Kai did not.

I was angry at this loss my son suffered so early on. I was angry at the Chinese government and his orphanage. I was incensed at the profound fallout on our family and its continued manifestation in our world. Persistent hypervigilance. Strained family relationships. Pent-up stress, leading to things like my climbing fall, or Scott's car accident that would happen five years later. The impact of Kai's early developmental losses never went away completely.

I began to realize that no amount of love would make up for the profound loss and abandonment Kai suffered. No amount of healing would recover what was absent in his earliest lonely years. No amount of knowledge or understanding would remedy the immense toll Kai's early neglect would take on my life and the life of our family. Like a dark, empty, leaking cavern, there would always be this hole in his soft, emotional center. We would need to learn how to abide with loss, to coexist with and welcome it as best we could. Loss would be with us for the foreseeable future.

SEEN AND HEARD

Each year, when summer ended and the kids were back in school, I was able to get together with a small group of other adoptive moms for lunch at a local Mexican restaurant. Two other moms in the group, Joan and Mary, had children from China, and both were forthright and honest about their struggles.

Mary was a retired physician who had recently sent her troubled son to a residential treatment facility somewhere in Montana after exhausting local therapists, schools, and treatment programs. She and her husband were fortunate enough to have had the financial means to send their son to reputable places, which specialize in treating children with histories of trauma and resulting attachment challenges. Her son Joey was twelve years old and had just started middle school. He had begun acting out physically against other students and had some of the same troubles I had always seen in Kai: sneakiness, food hoarding, stealing, and motivational challenges. We talked about how Reactive Attachment Disorder manifests itself as kids grow older, and we deliberated openly about whether or not Joey and Kai would ever grow out of their issues.

Mary and I were both exasperated with the amount of energy our sons took from us. Neither of us ever felt truly relaxed, always on edge when our boys were around. It was comforting talking to someone who intimately understood the life I was living. I felt affirmed and heard as I talked about how everything had changed since adopting our son— the chronic state of stress we lived in, the tiredness I always felt, and the obvious relationship it all had to my climbing accident, the fallout of which continued to have ramifications on our entire family.

"I don't know how you do it," Joan said to me, glancing over toward Mary and pointing at my crutches and ankle boot. "How long has this been going on? It has been over a year and a half, hasn't it?"

"I know," I responded. Sighing, I acknowledged that November would be the two-year anniversary of my climbing fall. "It's frustrating, trying to parent while trying to learn self-care. I've had so many surgeries and procedures. My doctors keep trying to fix this ankle, which is always throbbing and swollen. It takes so much out of me."

"I bet it does," Mary piped in. "It's not like our kids don't take enough out of us! What does your medical team recommend?"

"My foot and ankle doctor is suggesting either a fusion or an ankle replacement. I already had a bone graft, which took about six months to recover from. I'm having my doubts about either giving me back the quality of life I was used to."

I pulled my phone out of my purse, and brought up two pictures of my ankle, showing a detailed X-ray and CT scan.

"Your surgeon is telling you he can fix that?" Mary asked. "That bone defect on your CT scan is huge. I don't see any way they're going to be able to anchor a replacement joint on that. And with a fusion, they would need to probably take off at least an inch and a half of bone material before they could fuse it. That fusion would probably last five years before arthritis set in, and you'd need another fusion of the adjacent joints. Has your doctor talked about this with you?"

"Yeah," I shared. "I've already had ten surgeries—including a reconstruction, skin and bone grafts, wound debridements [also called 'washouts'] and lots of other limb-salvage procedures. None of these operations brought me any closer to having a non-painful, functional leg. I'm not excited about a future full of more surgeries. I'm tired of seeing myself as a patient. I'm beginning to wonder if amputation would be the best decision, even though it would be a hard one to make. I've seen happy-go-lucky below-knee amputees skipping along on their running blades, and I'm starting to wonder if I should just get off the limb-salvage treadmill and be done with it."

Mary looked at me over the top of her glasses, back down at the photos on my phone, and locked her gaze back onto mine once again.

"Orthopedics is a huge revenue generator in the healthcare industry," she owned. "It's a cash cow, and right now, you are a gold mine."

What Mary was sharing resonated with me. I had been gradually feeling less and less confident that I would ever regain my pre-accident quality of life, yet I kept covering my feelings of hopelessness and despair with the scraps of hope that my orthopedic team was throwing my way, smeared over with the thick balm of ever-present denial.

I peered back at Mary, my eyes bulging open wide. "Really? I'm a cash cow? Somehow that doesn't surprise me. I should have known."

"Look, I've worked in medicine for a long time, before it started becoming so corporate. I can certainly tell you about healthcare politics.

Surgeons are pressured to keep the OR full—because surgeries mean revenue. Insurance reimbursements for orthopedic surgeries are guaranteed profits for healthcare. It's an institution, like everything else these days." She shook her head, brushing crumbs off the table. "I hate to say it, but they're not going to tell you that amputation would be your best choice. That would be robbing them of the revenue they'd make off you with guaranteed future surgeries."

I realized that I should have been reeling back in sheer disgust as the conversation continued, but I wasn't. I relaxed my shoulders for once, beginning to feel the weight of denial being lifted and replaced with the validation I had been looking for. Deep down, I knew that the choice to move on to amputation was solely on me. I would need to keep asking the right questions and seeking the right answers.

"You're smart," Mary continued. "It's good that you're bringing up these questions now, and that you aren't afraid of going down that road. I have seen so many patients who didn't and they ended up having all kinds of other complications as a result of inactivity—obesity, diabetes, heart problems, depression. I know it's not easy, but you are doing the right thing. That ankle doesn't look fixable to me."

She went on to talk about a diabetic patient she had known who was depressed and despondent, knowing that he should probably undergo bilateral foot amputations to improve his circulation and ashen appearance. When he finally had the procedure, the color returned to his face, along with a new lust for life.

"You have houseplants, right?" she asked.

"Yes, of course."

"What do you do when the leaves begin to get brown and dry, or when the ends of the plant begin to die? You prune it! That gives the plant enough energy to continue growing again, without all its psychic energy going into the dying appendages. I think people are very similar."

"Wow, that is a great analogy!" I understood well the way my puffy, red, swollen foot drained my energy. Like a plant, I was physically and emotionally wilting from years of living with pain and debility creeping into my daily existence and camping out in my spirit. Remembering the levity felt by the amputees I met at the No Barriers Summit, I had already begun to conceptualize what life could be like if I made the difficult decision to amputate.

It would not be easy, but it would bring a certain degree of freedom. Life would look different, for sure. *Would amputation mean failure? Was I conceding?* I didn't think so. I had been tending to this dying append-age for longer than I had ever imagined I would, and I knew it was no longer serving me well. Coming up on two years, it was apparent that I was at a crossroads. Either way, I was looking down the road at a future where more pain and surgeries would be certain, but if I didn't make the decision to have an amputation, "recovery" would never end.

I had learned to adapt, knowing that my pelvic and lumbar disc fractures would likely mean lifelong lower back pain that I'd have to learn to manage. I longed to enjoy my family and my life despite these challenges. Sometimes you have to get rid of the things that drain you the most. I knew my throbbing, red angry ankle drained my life-force. It had to go.

TEN LITTLE PIGGIES

I've always been quite fond of my feet. When I was younger and my family would go on road trips, my sister Katie and I would be stuck in the back seat, bored and looking for something to do. We devised this strange game, "Good Foot, Bad Foot," giving anthropomorphic attributes to my right and left foot, respectively. Ah, the odd things fourth and sixth grade girls will do with too much time on their hands. We were very strange children.

Being right-side dominant, my right foot was more agile. Its toes were slightly angled and suction-cup-like, able to function oddly like fingers, which meant they could pick things up off the floor or hold an eating utensil. I joked that I had supremely talented feet, while Katie turned up her nose and assured me that my bony toes were quite ugly.

"Ewwww, I *hate* feet!" she would say, as I sneakily inched my powerful toes closer and closer to her across the brown vinyl back seat of my parent's Buick Skylark.

Over the years, my feet had served me very well in sports: my diving approach foot with an awesome toe point; my lead foot in coming out of the sprinting blocks in track; and my springy, leaping foot which piloted a formidable high jump.

In the summer as a young girl, I would run around barefoot from sunup to sundown, calluses conveniently hardening on the bottoms of my feet as I gingerly learned to navigate walking across the gravel street separating our house from the neighbor kids. I loved jumping rope in the smooth asphalt driveway and feeling the cool softness of the grass carpeting the backyard. My feet, including my ugly toes, were good to me.

Looking down upon my right foot and lower extremity in the wake of my accident, it was quite different. I was no longer able to point my toes down because my ankle could not bend in that way. The hunk of skin covering my ankle was rubbery and lacked tactile sensation. I had *maybe* ten degrees of plantar flexion and dorsiflexion when my foot wasn't pounding, inflamed, and swollen, at which time I would take to laying on the couch and elevating it. This existence was getting old.

I had wonderful memories of going barefoot on the beach, running through the water as a lifeguard, and jumping over the waves of North Beach in Lake Michigan. I knew these were comforting experiences which I could always cherish but would never experience again—with my current cobbled-together foot intact, or even potentially down the road as an amputee. I had been significantly, and irreversibly hobbled.

The longing to return to my pre-accident life continued to linger like a pesky bug I'd tried to shoo away with minimal success. I knew my spirit was dying on the vine. My non-functioning appendage needed to be pruned so my body could bounce back. Would I miss my right foot if I amputated? Of course. I already missed its functionality, and it now seemed pathetically foreign, unable to deliver its previous stellar abilities and ease of movement. I could not gain back the old "real" foot. I chose to focus on the people I'd met who embraced a mindset of adaptability alongside disability.

I began to realize that, with an amputation, my "disability" would be visible to all. Even though I had two intact legs, I felt more disabled than the amputees I had seen running by me at the No Barriers Summit. Would I be able to convince my surgeons that I wanted to get off the painful limb-salvage locomotive leading me to more guaranteed pain and suffering? I pondered what life would be like with limb loss and afterward, and I started talking with Scott and my family about the possibility of having a below knee amputation. I longed to reclaim my integrity as an active person and was ready to regain my quality of life. My family was too.

SECOND OPINION

Thanks to the internet, I had connected with a half dozen other people online who had incurred injuries similar to mine—a snowboarder, a skier, three rock climbers, and a marathon runner. All had suffered debilitating ankle fractures and undergone multiple surgeries over several years. Two had flown to a specialty hospital in New York City to have stem cells injected into their cartilage before being fitted with something called an "ilizarov frame"—a heavy Frankenstein-esque contraption resembling a ringed erector set, which would expand the joint space between the foot and ankle, with the hope of cartilage regrowth and healing. All three climbers decided to have below-knee amputations after realizing that their ankles would never be fixable (we had similar "mechanisms of injury"). The runner shared that she went through "twelve arduous years on the couch" before deciding to reclaim her life through amputation. She'd since started running again with a Cheetah blade, a prosthetic designed for the activity. Each of them gave me the same advice. Essentially: "Don't waste any more time. Your ankle is garbage. Lop the thing off."

I learned that "elective amputation" was not something that was taken lightly by the orthopedic community. "Once you cut your leg off, you can't change your mind" was a common refrain.

My foot and ankle doctor assured me that his soccer coach ran quite well after an ankle fusion. While I took this into consideration, I also began asking others with the same mechanism of injury that I had about their experiences. Three fellow climbers had endured several fusions, which were incredibly painful, and had ended up amputating anyway. Two had attempted ankle replacement surgeries, which failed. The sentiment was unanimous: *your life is precious. Don't waste your time trying to fix the unfixable.*

I set up an appointment for a second opinion with a specialist who worked for a different medical group on the opposite side of town. Dr. Gifford was a seasoned orthopedic surgeon who was also a tenured instructor at the Medical College, someone I felt confident had seen many severe cases such as mine.

"Hi, I'm Dr. Gifford," he said as he walked in, extending his hand. "I hear you are here for a second opinion. What happened that you fractured your ankle? How long has it been? I see you are still in the boot."

I told him about my 30-foot climbing fall, along with additional details regarding my spinal and pelvic fracture and sacroiliac joint fusion.

"It's coming up on two years that we've been trying to fix this thing. I had the external fixator, the reconstruction surgery, a free flap, a bone graft, hardware removal. The list goes on."

"Wow. Sounds like you really did a number on your ankle," he responded. "I'd be happy to look at your X-rays. Did you bring them with you today?"

I opened the manilla file folder, took out two envelopes containing the DVDs of my X-rays and CT scans, and handed them over.

"Wonderful," he said. "I'll just take a quick look at these while you take your boot off."

I watched as Dr. Gifford slid the DVD into the reading device and pulled the scans up on the computer screen before sitting in the chair next to the examination table. The four Velcro straps made a ripping noise as I pulled them back and removed the heavy boot, setting it next to my chair. The toes protruding from my bandaged foot were starting to become red and puffy because my leg had been dangling down, and I had been sitting with my foot at floor level, letting the blood pool in my throbbing lower extremity. This was what happened whenever I wasn't able to elevate it. Slowly, I unwrapped the ACE bandage, then hoisted my foot up on the examination table.

Dr. Gifford looked back from his computer screen and rolled his chair closer to me, leaning in to look at my unbandaged ankle. "When was your accident?"

"It was November, coming up on two years ago."

"The free flap looks good. How far are you able to walk on it?"

"Not far at all. I wear the boot and usually bring crutches because it hurts to bear any weight on my ankle."

"Mmmm. I can see that," he responded, before turning back around to look at the computer screen. I watched as he clicked between various images of my ankle. It was eerily quiet as he leaned in toward the monitor for what felt like ten minutes or more, examining the different angles of my ankle images. I remained silent, not wanting to disturb whatever was going on in his head.

Dr. Gifford nodded three deep nods before quickly shaking his head from side to side and spinning his chair around. He wheeled back to my direction once again. Pressing his fingers together, he looked at me squarely and stated, "You realize that you basically demolished your ankle joint. It really doesn't get much more severe than this."

"Yeah, I know." I chuckled nervously, looking down at the floor and back at the good doctor. "That's why I'm here. I don't think there is much more that can be done to give me my life back. I've always been an active person. I miss it."

An unexpected reaction spread across Dr. Gifford's face, surprising me. It appeared to be anger or disgust, which I did not understand. I waited to see what was coming, somewhat fearful about what I would hear.

He sighed deeply once again, pressing his hands together and under his chin. He looked straight at me and said, "These young doctors. They want to be big shots, going to their conferences and promoting their work. I know how this goes. I've been there."

I listened intently, but I wasn't quite sure where this conversation was going. I had a hunch that he probably knew my previous surgeon from the Medical College. He'd probably even taught him at some point. Clearly, the sentiments he was sharing were not directed at me. They were directed at my previous doctor.

"Look," he continued. "There is *no way in hell* a replacement joint would ever anchor into that tremendous bone defect." With a pen, he pointed to the darkened inch-and-a-half area at the bottom of my tibia on the X-ray. "You see all this area? No amount of bone graft material will make it workable. I think you've just been wasting your time."

My heart sank. "Wasting my time? You're basically saying that the last year and a half, I have been hobbling around for nothing? There was no hope of healing?"

Dr. Gifford paused for a moment, and said, "Basically, yes."

I was flooded with a mixture of anger, relief, and fear. Anger at my previous surgeon for leading me on and promising false hope, relief in gaining affirmation of what I knew in my heart, and fear of not knowing what he would propose for my next steps. I knew I was ready to move on to amputation, even though I realized these conversations were serious and tricky.

"What would you recommend at this point?" I asked.

"If you were to have a fusion, you would lose at least an inch and a half of leg length on your right side. That bone defect is not workable, even for a fusion."

I had done my homework and learned about something called the "kinetic chain"—the interrelationship between all the body's joints, working together in alignment with the spine to create optimal function and balance.

"You know, my back is already jacked from my sacroiliac joint fusion. Adding a limb-length discrepancy would be horrible for my back. Plus, putting an inch-and-a-half lift on my shoe seems like a suboptimal solution for a highly active person."

He looked at my X-ray on the computer screen again, and then clicked back over to the CT scan. He peered back to me once more.

"You know there is only one other option other than a fusion here, right?" He had to know I had considered amputation, but I knew providers could not take these conversations lightly. They were probably as difficult as discussing any end-stage disease or the kinds of options that seemed like giving up.

"I *have* thought about amputation," I owned up. "I've been in touch with lots of other people who had similar kinds of fractures. I've seen people do just fine with prosthetics. If that is what you would recommend, I'd be ready for it."

Dr. Gifford was quiet for a moment. I knew he was part of a medical system that often equated amputation with giving up. A failure to "fix" the problem. He also seemed to be seasoned enough to know that the system sometimes fails its patients, that often there are no optimal solutions.

"Yes, amputation would be an option," he finally conceded. "There are good prosthetics out there these days, which could definitely give you a better quality of life than you have now."

I began to feel a twinge of relief.

"But obviously, there is no turning back. It's a done deal. You can't put it back on."

I thought, *Here we go again with the "You can't tape your leg back on" scenario. Puhleeze. As if I hadn't considered this already.*

"These kinds of fractures—pilon fractures from a fall from a height—are always the ones that make us cringe. There are no good ways of fixing them. Maybe someday the technology will be better in the field, but right now, it's not. Not for ankles like this, anyway. It's up to you. A fusion would buy you more time, but you would probably end up having an amputation down the road anyway. Neither option is a good one. I'm sorry," he concluded.

"You're not telling me anything I wasn't prepared for," I responded. "I have two young children and am ready to do whatever it takes to get my life back."

Dr. Gifford shook his head again. "I'm just sorry that your previous doctor put you through this. I can't in good faith tell you that we can fix this ankle with a replacement joint. If you had been seeing me, I would have been more honest from the get-go. It would be a setup for failure. Keep in touch and let me know what you decide. Good luck."

Dr. Gifford and I shook hands again. He assured me that he would continue to be available for consultation if I needed more advice. I had gained a helpful, alternative perspective about my situation, along with an interesting window into the world of orthopedic politics.

THIRD OPINION

As I began to think more seriously about amputation, I learned that it would be a good idea to attend an amputee peer support group in my area to ask questions of people who were living with limb loss. Obviously, the big black orthopedic boot would be a glaring clue that I was not yet in the limb loss club, but I was ready to explain that I was considering becoming a card-carrying member.

An older gentleman named Al approached me as I entered the door. Al was a friendly below-knee amputee who I'd guessed to be around age 70. He introduced himself and began asking me questions.

"I see you're wearing a boot. Let me guess, you're considering amputation?"

"Yes," I acknowledged. "I've been trying to save this thing for going on two years now. I thought maybe the group would have some good advice for me." I pointed at my ankle with an annoyance that was only partially in jest.

"You know," Al responded. "It's an expensive club to be in. It'll cost you an arm and a leg, for sure."

I laughed and slapped my knee, acknowledging the beauty of amputee humor.

"Five years ago, I was in the same boat you're in," Al shared. "I was in a car accident, and I had surgery after surgery to try to fix it. I gained a ton of weight. Finally, my wife suggested we get a second opinion, and by that time, infection had set in. I didn't have a choice."

"How did you adjust?" I asked, "Did you ever have any regrets?"

"None whatsoever," Al responded. "Other than the fact that I wish I would have done it sooner. The amputation was way easier than all the other surgeries—and much less painful! Don't get me wrong, it's an adjustment. You need to find a good prosthetist, like I did. Not all of them are good, but they're out there."

I learned that, like most medical situations, the prosthetic industry is a business and the more knowledge I could gain about it, the better.

"Do you have a surgeon in mind to discuss amputation with?" Al asked, pouring himself a cup of coffee and grabbing a napkin.

"No, not yet. I probably should ask around to find out who would be reputable doctor to see."

"I had Dr. Harris do my amputation, and I can't recommend him highly enough." Al opened his wallet and handed me Dr. Harris' business card. Dr. Harris was affiliated with the same hospital and medical center I had already been involved with! He hadn't been on my team as his specialization had him located in a different office. It would certainly be worth a try chatting with him. "You should call him. If and when you see him, tell him I say hello and that I'm doing well."

"Thanks, I will!" I said. "You have been so helpful." I felt an instant surge of excitement that I had found a connection and possible solution to my current, painful, limb-salvage situation.

The rest of the peer support meeting went well. I met several arm amputees—two had lost their arms in farming accidents, unfortunately quite common here in the Midwest. Two men had above-knee amputations and discussed their problems with the new bionic knee technology and insurance. "BKAs [below-knee amputees] are lucky to not need a prosthetic knee, so the issues are not quite as complicated," I was told.

As I left the meeting, I felt confident that I had learned a great deal. I had obtained a referral of a doctor to potential do the amputation, and I had spoken with others who were living with limb loss and thriving.

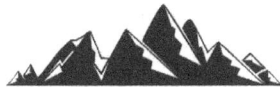

I called Dr. Harris' office and was fortunate to obtain an appointment only two weeks out. When speaking with the scheduler, I assured her that all my records could be obtained from the previous appointments and hospitalizations I had, as they were in the same medical system. I told her that I wanted to consult with Dr. Harris about a possible amputation surgery, that I had suffered through nearly two years of limb-salvage surgeries and was ready to talk about other options. I listened to her typing on the keyboard as she collected all the necessary information. Scott agreed to take the day off to accompany me to the appointment. I wanted back up to make sure I didn't forget any important details.

Dr. Harris walked into the room accompanied by his female physician assistant and nurse. He wore outmoded glasses, was balding and, surprisingly, even shorter than my husband. Dr. Harris introduced himself and his team members; the former carried a file folder and the latter stood in the corner of the room, silently nodding. They both remained standing, while Dr. Harris leaned against the countertop.

"What is it you're here for?" Dr. Harris asked, looking between Scott and me. "I have seen your images. I know that you've had quite a few operations. That's quite a fracture you suffered!"

I was glad that he had already seen the images of my ankle, and I had a hunch that he had already spoken to my foot and ankle surgeon. I got an odd vibe from the dynamics I was see between the doctor and his subordinates. It was obvious he was used to having a certain degree of power. The two women appeared to be comfortable being more subservient and remaining in the background.

"I'm glad that you saw my images," I responded. "You know that I've been at this game for almost two years. I've done my homework. I know there is nothing else that can be done to give me the quality of life I want—other than amputation. I have always been an athlete. I'm an active person, and I can do more with a prosthetic leg than I can with this painful, useless, cobbled-together ankle."

Dr. Harris bent his elbow and supported his chin with his hand, bending finger over his mouth and nodding. He remained quiet, so I continued.

"I have two young kids. I miss running around and playing with them. I miss not being in pain all the time. I'm tired of lugging along this ankle boot and constantly elevating my foot because of the swelling and puffiness. Again, it has been almost two years! I'm done. I'm ready to have it taken off!"

Dr. Harris looked at the physician assistant, then back to me and Scott. I glanced sideways at Scott, who was sitting next to me on the blue examination table.

He piped up. "Yeah, I can attest that it has been a pretty miserable two years. All the surgeries, the pain medications, the hospitalizations. She's ready to move on. We all are."

The silent nurse walked over from the corner of the room and stood next to Dr. Harris. I was surprised when she began to speak.

"Amputation is hard," she said. "There are prosthetic fitting problems. Insurance hassles. Healing issues. It's not that easy. We had a patient just yesterday whose insurance denied a claim to get a prosthetic leg. Insurance hassles are real and they're tough to deal with."

I bristled for a moment. Was this woman minimizing my decision to do something about these very real, life-changing, painful issues because she saw the temporary challenges and inconveniences that *might happen* as a real problem?

"I know about these things," I responded. "Again, I have done my homework. I've talked to a lot of folks who have been in my position. I know about insurance hassles and, thank God, I'm a former social worker with a good understanding of how to get through to insurance companies. It's not like I haven't thought long and hard about this."

Dr. Harris chuckled briefly in a low tone. "When your leg is gone, it's not like we can reattach it again." He looked to Scott, as if my husband would understand something I didn't.

Again, no shit, I thought.

"Have you talked with your ankle doctor about fusion?" Dr. Harris added.

I was beginning to feel increasingly irritated and frustrated, yet I knew that I needed to give the complete lowdown again.

"Yes. Did you notice from my records that I also have a right SI joint fusion? My spinal fractures and SI joint are important factors here. A near two-inch limb-length discrepancy and a generally immobile foot would be horrible for my back. At least prosthetic feet have some bounce, and I can be sure my back, hips, and pelvis are in alignment."

The nurse piped up again. "Nothing can prepare you for waking up after anesthesia and looking down to notice your leg is gone. Amputation is a loss. I've been in the OR during many amputations. It truly feels like a death in that room."

Momentarily, I felt empathy for the staff in the room with me. "That must be very hard for you."

"It is," she said. "It is very quiet in there. Very somber."

My empathy turned to simmering indignation as I began to realize it was not my role to provide empathy to the medical professionals assigned to my case. It was their job to listen and be compassionate to my needs. It was their role to partner with me and gain an understanding of what would serve me best in my quest to regain my quality of life.

I swallowed my anger and attempted to soften the discussion with a bit of humor. "Oh, I wouldn't know. I'm never awake when I'm in the operating room,"

Scott began to see and feel the same dynamics and unacknowledged pushback from these three medical folks that I did.

"Look," Scott said. "I've never known Chris to be this unhappy. Being active—hiking, running, climbing, biking—those things are a big part of who she is. She has talked to people in her very same situation, and all of them have said they wish they would have amputated earlier."

Dr. Harris nodded his head and picked up my medical file from the countertop. "Let me give this all some thought. I will get back to you in a couple of weeks." He walked over to shake Scott's hand, then mine, before filing out of the room. His nurse and physician assistant followed closely behind.

I felt defeated, unheard, and angry. The way he'd acted confirmed my suspicions that Dr. Harris had likely consulted with my previous surgeon beforehand and had already made up his mind prior to meeting with us. I remembered my conversation at lunch with Mary about orthopedics being a cash cow for hospital revenue. There was no way in hell I was going to defer to this man's allegiance to the system or his team's apparent feelings of "death-like sadness and loss" in the operating room. Determined not to give my power away, I resolved to pursue three additional opinions. I maneuvered on my knee scooter to the medical records office to sign off on getting my medical documentation and getting out of there.

I fantasized about calling Dr. Harris and talking with his staff about the emotional maturity that comes with living with loss, of moving through loss and integrating it. I wondered if the trauma of their jobs had jaded them to the potential growth that could come through loss, and the depth that could be gained. I felt confident in myself and proud of the physical, spiritual, and emotional work I had done up until that point. I was more than ready to move on.

FOURTH, FIFTH, AND SIXTH OPINIONS

The amputee community is chock-full of strong, gnarly, survivor types. Having to navigate life after limb-loss seems to render folks quite creative and scrappy. Through this network, I garnered three additional medical opinions from top-notch surgeons in the field of foot and ankle surgery. One was from Georgetown University Hospital in D.C., another was from the Limb Preservation Institute in Denver, Colorado, and the last was from Oklahoma University Medical Center. All were highly specialized in working with complex cases such as mine.

I sent each of these surgeons my huge stack of medical records, knowing that it might take some time for them to read through it all. I didn't care. I wanted to be sure I exhausted all my options and received the best possible advice.

Within a month's time, I had received a personal phone call from each doctor. Each one was forthright in his belief that no further surgical option could give me a better quality of life than amputation. Each surgeon began the conversation by acknowledging that I had obliterated my ankle beyond repair and apologized for the two years of hell I had lived through in attempts to salvage this unfixable limb.

The Georgetown doctor phoned first, on a Tuesday evening. "Wow," he began "You did a number on your ankle. There's no good way to fix it, and I'm sorry—but it sounds like you've come to the place of literally wanting to cut your losses, yes?" Relieved that he understood my situation, I admitted that I was ready to do whatever it would take to regain my active lifestyle. "I've seen so many people in your situation make the decision to have a below-knee amputation," he continued. "They regain their lives, move on with their new normal, and they never look back. I'm glad to see you're at this point. You've got the grit and the right attitude. I know you'll do great!"

I spoke to the doctor from Denver next. "Look, I love my job," the surgeon shared. "I love to salvage limbs, lengthen limbs, surgically fix them in any way possible. I find the carpentry and architecture of bodies fascinating. When I have a patient or family come to me and want me to do everything I can to save their limb, I'm happy to. But I've also worked with many people such as yourself—many of them climbers actually—and I can honestly look them in the eye and tell them that a good prosthetic will give you much more than limb-salvage can. There is no way my fixing your limb will give you the quality of life that you're looking for. But a prosthetic device can."

I was so grateful for this doctor's honesty—not only regarding my situation, but also in response to the medical model of "fixing."

The humility that came through in his conversation with me was something I had been deeply craving all along. I felt like he actually cared. I was not an injury to be fixed, but a *person* with a life on hold, longing to be active again. We spoke for about 45 minutes before hanging up. I thanked him for taking the time to weed through my medical records and getting back to me about this life-changing decision. He was genuinely happy to do so.

The third and final doctor to review my records and get back to me was the one from OU Medical. Dr. William Ertl was a relatively young and hip orthopedic surgeon, whose grandfather had actually developed an amputation bone-bridge procedure while fixing up American soldiers in Germany during World War II. Dealing with soldiers' losing limbs during the war, he recognized that they were often left with great pain and disability following limb loss, because not enough attention to detail was taken to bury nerve endings within muscle and create a stable, weight-bearing residual limb. Many amputees suffered from horrible phantom limb pain. He created a specialized technique to help eliminate these problems, the eponymous "Ertl osteomyoplastic amputation."

"I looked through all of your medical records Chris," Dr. Ertl said as our phone call began. "And there were a lot of them. I'm an orthopedic surgeon, so this is what I do. I like to look at the whole person, not just the ankle—which, in your case, is basically destroyed. How long has it been? Almost two years or so?"

"Yeah, two long years," I responded. "I'm so tired of lugging around this painful ankle."

"I bet you are. This was from a climbing fall?"

"Yup. I fell about 30 feet or so. Big brain fart—forgot to clip into the auto belay at the gym. Fractured my L1, L4, and L5, my S1, and my pelvis, too. Did you see that in my records?"

"Yup, I did. Boy, you really did a number on your body, especially your ankle. I'm sorry that this happened, and that your recovery seems to have been really hard."

"Oh yeah." I admitted to the pain, disability, and frustrations with my medical team, which had lead to feelings of hopelessness, often bordered on despair. "It has become more and more challenging as time has gone on."

"And your doctors have wanted to do an ankle replacement or a fusion, right? I see these cases a lot, maybe not even as severe as yours. I wouldn't even think about fusing your ankle. The bone stock is horrible and you would lose significant limb length. That would be really bad for the alignment of your back and pelvis."

Finally, I thought. A surgeon who saw me as a whole person, not just someone with an appendage to be fixed. I breathed a sigh of relief into the phone. "I can't believe you just said that. I've been trying to convince my doctor here of all these issues being related, but I was always brushed aside."

Dr. Ertl responded. "I can tell you've done your homework. You're smart. I can also tell you that, without a doubt, after the initial few months post-amputation, you'll begin to get your active life back. The prosthetic fitting process will take some time. The first year is always the hardest, but it won't even be as hard as what you've been through already."

"What about potential complications?" I asked. "Infection, non-healing bone problems, fit issues…"

"You're otherwise very healthy," he replied. "You're relatively young and active. No diabetes. No circulation problems. You don't smoke. I don't foresee any complications, other than needing to have a good degree of patience with the healing and prosthetic fitting process."

We continued our long conversation about what it would take to move forward with the procedure. "You've literally done hundreds of these, right?"

"Probably more than that," he responded. "I'm one of a handful of surgeons who is able to see amputation as a potential step in the right direction, because I've seen firsthand the benefits of prosthetic technology.

As surgeons, we can't fix everything. I even have a prosthetist and a physical therapist in the operating room with me when I'm performing the procedure to consult with, just to make sure we are taking everything into consideration with build-height and feet down the road. I like to work as a team."

This sounded fantastic to me. I loved the fact that Dr. Ertl collaborated with other disciplines in his role. It gave me confidence that he didn't have some type of God complex or huge ego. I was increasingly inclined to travel to Oklahoma to have the amputation done by Dr. Ertl.

"I'll need to talk to my husband," I said, "but do you think we would be able to fly down there to have you do the surgery?"

"People fly here all the time. I can have my administrative assistant get back to you with details, but I could probably get you on the surgery schedule sometime in January. I have all the information I need from your records, and I would just need to see you in my office a few days beforehand for a pre-surgical visit and some lab work."

It all sounded good to me, and I began to feel a twinge of relief and hope returning, after almost two years of setbacks, frustration, and heartache. I was grateful to finally feel understood and valued. My integrity was not linked to the success of a surgery or achieving a medical goal, but to the triumph of my spirit and ability to overcome all of the obstacles thrown in my direction.

I didn't see the loss of a limb as a failure but as a bridge to a new and exciting life chapter. My wilting, weary spirit perked up again for the first time in a very long while, and I began to feel alive again.

I phoned Dr. Ertl's office and spoke to the administrative assistant.

"I'm ready to schedule my amputation. Is it weird that I'm excited?"

"Not at all," she responded. "We hear that a lot. Most folks like you go through years of hell before they decide to come here. You're lucky it's only been two years. You haven't had the cumulative effect of weight gain, depression, diabetes, or other problems that arise after years of inactivity."

We planned to celebrate my last two-footed holiday season with the family before flying down to Oklahoma City for my amputation, which was scheduled for the second week of January 2013.

"So you'll be kind of like a robot mom? Will you still be able to climb?" Jade asked, after we told the kids.

"Yes, honey," I replied. "I'll need different legs for different activities, but I'll still be able to climb."

"What about the beach?" she asked.

"The beach?" Kai echoed, gesturing with his hands as if to swim the front crawl.

I sighed, aware that water sports and activities tended to be a pain with prosthetic componentry.

"We'll have to see, Kai. We'll have to see."

AMPUTATION

Getting organized for my amputation surgery was no small feat. I had to prepare for two months of downtime upon my return from Oklahoma. We had to plan our trip and organize all the details. I needed to square away all the insurance paperwork ahead of time and set up an initial appointment with a prosthetist back home to start a relationship in preparation for having a prosthetic leg made.

The kids would return to school after the holidays. We needed to find someone to stay with them while Scott and I traveled to Oklahoma. Scott's brother Matt (a grad student at the time), had winter break that week, and we were thankful that he offered up to move into our house for the week to take care of Jade, Kai, and our cats. He was a fun and loving, no-nonsense uncle with a keen awareness of Kai's dynamics, not afraid to put the smack down if necessary. He had been with us previously on a trip to Devil's Lake State Park as a babysitter for Kai while Scott and I took a course in setting up ropes for climbing.

He agreed to wake Jade and Kai up each morning, make their lunches, feed them breakfast, and get them out the door for school on time. He also stayed on top of the kids' homework and remained connected with their teachers while we were obviously preoccupied. We were fortunate that Uncle Matt could fill this very important role for us while we were away. With the utmost confidence in Matt, we entrusted our children to him for the week, and set off.

We arrived in Oklahoma City late on a Monday evening, with the plan to go to my pre-op appointment early the next day. Matt and the kids called to video chat one last time before I was to go under the knife. They were curious and excited to talk.

"Mom, are you scared to get your leg cut off?" Jade asked.

"No, not really, honey," I responded. "You know about all those other surgeries I had. Those were probably even longer and harder than this one will be."

"Really?" The kids seemed surprised that I wasn't afraid.

I recalled the comment Dr. Harris' nurse made: "Nothing can prepare you for waking up after anesthesia and seeing that your leg is gone," and I wondered if I would feel this way. I doubted it. I was so ready to have this worthless appendage gone.

The following morning, we arrived at Dr. Ertl's office, where we also met the doctor of physical therapy, physician assistant, and a prosthetist who would be present during the amputation. I was able to ask lots of last-minute questions about prosthetics and the adjustment to life as an amputee.

"What will happen with my leg remains?" I asked.

"It's protocol to send it to pathology before it goes to the incinerator," Dr. Ertl's PA shared. "Unless you request to have something else done with it. There is a taxidermist in town that some patients have sent their remains to, and they do a pretty good job of preserving the bones."

"*Really?*" I couldn't believe a business would do this type of thing with *human* remains. I was slightly intrigued, as I was curious about the three-dimensional architecture of my damaged ankle. But the ick factor strongly superseded my curiosity. "I'll pass on that. The incinerator will be just fine, thanks."

Dr. Ertl and his staff all expressed hope and excitement for what I would regain after amputation. They had seen many patients like me and knew that this would be the catalyst for getting my life back. I felt confident and reassured to have upbeat, positive folks in my court who saw the potential of a full life after limb loss, as opposed to viewing this as some horrible mourning experience.

"You will do so well. I'm excited for you," Dr. Ertl said.

The following morning was show time. Scott and I woke up at 5:00 a.m. and presented ourselves to the hospital admissions desk at 5:45. I was taken to the pre-op area and given a hospital gown to change into before the medical assistant returned with a little jar in hand. "You know how this goes. We need a urine sample for a pregnancy test. It's just protocol."

"Ha. I'm 45 and I'm sure I'm not pregnant, but okay." I took the cup and hobbled to the bathroom at the end of the hallway.

As discussed, I knew I would once again have an epidural before the surgery. I was not excited about this but knew I would be grateful for it after the amputation. It was a painful procedure, but worth it for its ability to keep my brain from registering the pain. The pain management team came into my room to discuss the procedure briefly, saying they were waiting for the thumbs up from the lab. The plan was to place the epidural at 7:00 a.m.

Scott and I waited, talking back and forth about how crazy and frustrating this journey had been. We joked about the strangeness of being excited to get my leg chopped off. Seven o'clock came and went, and we continued to wait for the pain management team. "I wish they'd shake a leg!" I chortled.

The head of the pain management team came into my room at 7:25 a.m., sighing. "Your pregnancy test came back positive."

"*What?!*" Scott and I were both aghast. There was no way in hell I could be pregnant, I was completely sure. My plumbing had never worked. I had an IUD placed to help with heavy menstrual flow shortly after my accident. *Could it have fallen out or malfunctioned?* I wondered. Still, Scott and I weren't young rabbits anymore. The likelihood of my being pregnant was virtually nil.

"I'm sure that I'm not pregnant. Is there a possibility that it could be a false positive?" I asked. "Could we repeat the test?"

"Sure," the staff member said. "This happens sometimes. We'll do a blood test this time just to be sure. We can't go ahead with the procedure until we are absolutely sure you aren't pregnant. It's part of our medical oath to do no harm."

Next, an anesthesiologist and her team came into the room and introduced themselves before placing an IV in my left arm, to be left in place during the surgery. Blood was also drawn for the repeat pregnancy test, and we were informed that we would have to wait, likely for another 30 minutes, for the lab to read the results.

I was nervous. There was a time when we sincerely hoped for pregnancy to happen. This was *not* one of those moments. We had our children, and our plates were full.

"Wouldn't *that* be something—we travel all this way to have my leg cut off, only to be denied the surgery because we're having a baby?" I blurted to Scott, who was patiently sitting against the wall. He laughed and joined me in considering the feasible of pregnancy. We both knew that there was really no way. Maybe a 0.005 percent chance.

Dr. Ertl came in with the pain management team at eight o'clock, giving a thumbs up.

"The test came back negative, so we're good to go," the pain team confirmed.

"Thank God!" I exclaimed, letting out a sigh of relief. "I was pretty sure I wasn't, but I was still sweating bullets until you got here!"

I was asked to lay on my side while the team placed the epidural into my back—I was ready for the poke and the burn. When the injection was done, Scott and I kissed and gave a sideways hug as the team announced that we were ready to proceed with the surgery. We were already behind schedule. A tear rolled down my cheek.

"You got this." Scott said, kissing me on the forehead.

"I know. It's just emotional. Give my best to the kids. Tell them I'm okay. Love you! See you on the other side."

The team wheeled me into the operating room, where Dr. Ertl greeted me wearing his bright blue scrubs and skull cap. "Are you doing okay? Are we ready for this?"

The morning had already been more eventful than I had preferred. I was more nervous than I had anticipated. "I guess," I answered. My voice was shallow and slightly shaky. I knew the days ahead would not be easy, but I was prepared for this.

The epidural was working. I felt numb below my belly button. A feeling of relaxation began to come over me, and I knew that I had probably been given a benzo to assist in calming me down for the surgery. Dr. Ertl stood at my left side with an oxygen mask in hand. IV meds were running through my veins. "Okay, here we go. Breathe deeply," he said, placing the mask over my nose and mouth.

I breathed in and surrendered my trust to Dr. Ertl in his medical team, feeling hopeful for my recovery and the days and weeks ahead.

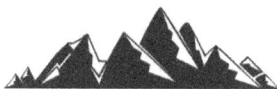

I woke up after the surgery in a groggy haze and immediately looked down at my leg. The nurse beside me was typing at her computer.

"How are you doing, Chris?" she asked. I noticed her white pearl nail polish as she fastened the blood pressure cuff on my arm to get my vitals.

"I'm okay," I responded. "Just wanted to look down to make sure my leg was really gone—and it is." I exhaled a sense of relief and gave her the cliff-note version of my accident and leg saga.

"Wow, that's crazy," she responded. "Dr. Ertl is great. You're in good hands."

I did not feel any sense of mourning or loss as Dr. Harris' nurse had warned; I felt a huge sense of relief! Finally, I was rid of this painful part of my life that had held me back for so long. I saw my white, delicately bandaged nub—or "stump," as "residual limbs" are affectionately called in the amputee world—laying on top of the light blue hospital blanket and felt no pain.

I was grateful that the epidural was still doing its job. I continued to feel no pain, only a little wooziness from the anesthesia. A sticky transdermal patch was applied to the curved part of my neck behind my left ear to administer medication to help with post-anesthesia nausea. Dr. Ertl's physician assistant approached the side of my bed and informed me that the surgery went well.

"Scott is waiting upstairs in your room for you. We will leave the epidural in for a few days to help with the pain. Let us know if the nausea gets worse and we can give you some more medication, okay?"

I proceeded to do just fine and was wheeled to my hospital room. Scott had been nodding off in the chair next to the bed but awakened quickly when we entered the room.

"Well, sounds like everything went well," he said, looking down at my amputated limb.

"Yup. And I looked down at my missing leg and felt relief. Not grief or loss, as Dr. Harris' staff warned."

Scott shook his head and came over to give me a kiss. "Glad it went well. I called the kids, and they are looking forward to hearing from you."

I dozed on and off for the next day or so, allowing the epidural to do its job. My pain was kept at bay until the third day of my hospitalization, when the epidural had to be removed. I knew this pain would be significant yet temporary. I was thankful for the pain medication which helped curb the intense hot throbbing I felt in my amputated leg. It helped to keep it elevated.

On the fourth day after the amputation, the physical therapist came into my room with a silver walker. "We're getting you up and about today. Hopefully you'll get to leave tomorrow. We'll see."

I pivoted to the side of the bed, keeping my nub as elevated as I could. It hurt when my leg hung down. The hot, searing rush of blood to the severed area was intense.

"Yeow! It's painful!" I exclaimed, gritting my teeth and grabbing the bars of the walker with stiff arms to remain upright. I knew it would take six to eight weeks for my nub to heal enough to be fitted for a prosthetic leg. Luckily, I was agile and fit enough to figure out maneuvering with whatever durable medical equipment I would have to use for the time being. Crutches, wheelchair, walker, or whatever.

"I know. That will go away. I promise," the PT assured.

Dr. Ertl came to my room wearing his business clothes as I made my way back to my bed. "Looks like you're doing great!" he said. "I think we will send you home tomorrow. I've got you set up this afternoon for an appointment at my office to get you cleared to fly home. We'll get you a plastic leg protector—you'll need it for your travels."

The final appointment went swimmingly. Dr. Ertl gave me a final thumbs up. "All looks good!"

I called the kids on the phone to touch base that evening. "Guess what? I'm coming home tomorrow! I'm so excited to see you guys!"

Uncle Matt put the phone on speaker to let the kids talk.

"I miss you," Jade said. "We're looking forward to have you back home!"

Kai grabbed the phone and asked to talk. "I love you, Mom. I miss you!"

Wow! I was surprised. This wasn't Kai's norm to tell me he missed me.

"I love and miss you too, Kai!" I responded, wondering if absence had made Kai's heart grow fonder.

Uncle Matt shared that he was very tired. "This parenting thing is a helluva lot of work!"

We laughed, knowing full well the all-in effort that parenting our children would be. We were so appreciative of Matt for helping us out in this way.

"How have the kids been?" I asked.

"Well, you know your son." Matt responded. "Put it this way, I'm glad I could send them to school. When he was home, I kept a tight eye on him."

I could tell by the interaction on the other end of the phone that this had been a sort of bonding experience for Matt and the kids (Kai always connected better with males), and I was thankful that everything had worked out so well. We were damned lucky. I was relieved, proud we were over the hump of this intense, excruciating ordeal, and ready to be back home.

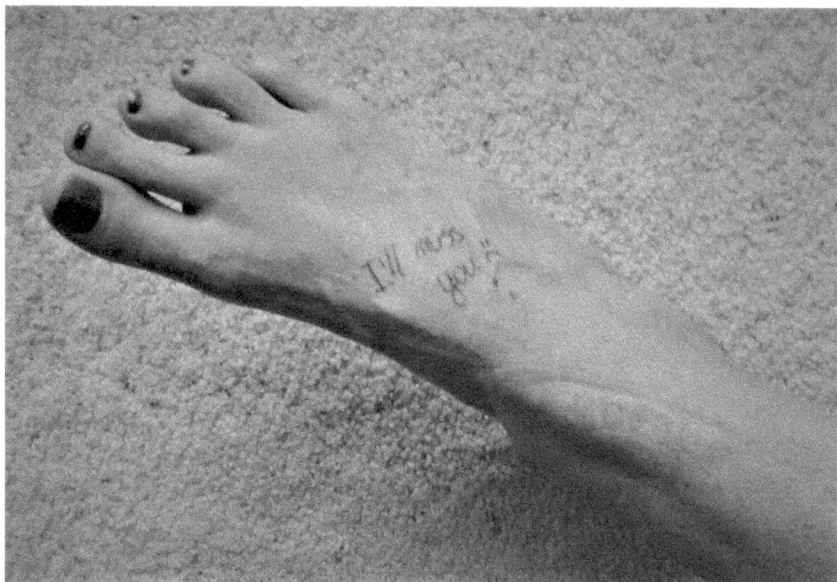

Pre–amputation foot farewell, 2013.

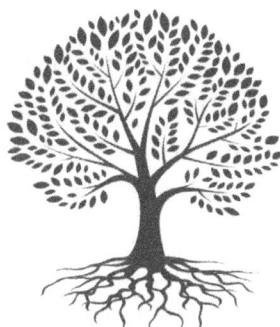

CHAPTER 6

HOBBLED AND WHOLE

NEW LIMITATIONS

Scott and I returned from Oklahoma City late Sunday evening, welcomed home by the kids, Uncle Matt, and my folks. They all were curious to find out how things went with my amputation.

"Do you feel like your leg is still there?"

"Are you in pain?"

"Has it been hard to wrap your head around your foot being gone?"

While there was some degree of pain, the worst of it had subsided at the hospital in the couple of days after the epidural wore off. I used a knee scooter to traverse the main floor of our house, a wheelchair to maneuver on longer trips out of the house for shopping and medical appointments, and a pair of crutches to hobble around the bedrooms and bathroom upstairs. When navigating the steps, I was shameless and crawled. My knees worked just fine and were more stable than trying to negotiate a couple of unwieldy crutches on stairs. The kids tried to help by taking their own laundry up and down the stairs of our tri-level house and cleaning the cat litter boxes in the basement. They learned how to throw their own wet snow clothes in the dryer, clear the table after dinner, and empty and load the dishwasher. Bonus!

I needed to take it easy for the six weeks after returning home, and was forced to re-learn the delicate art of self-compassion (by now, an ongoing lesson). This meant I had to delegate many tasks to others, including Jade and Kai, readjust my expectations, and learn to accept help more often. All of this became more and more second-nature as the months wore on, but it was a hard transition to make. I felt a compelled to bounce back as quickly as possible and prove I could still tackle life head-on. Obviously, this change required patience, including learning to walk on a prosthetic leg.

The process for making the prosthetic leg took time. First, insurance authorization was needed, which was problematic because my insurance company decided to be difficult and require mountains of documentation to prove I would use a prosthetic leg well. Once approved, the prosthetist made a see-through plastic "check-socket" that could be modified before creating the finished, carbon fiber leg. Everyone watched as I gingerly took my first few steps between the long, silver bars.

My first steps in a prosthetic leg felt strange. Not painful, just different. Rolling a gel liner on my nub felt a bit like getting used to wearing a bra: I didn't like it, but knew it was necessary, and I learned about the importance of a fit that was snug but not too snug. Over time I learned that adding socks of varying plies created an optimal fit.

Ambulating felt a bit like walking in a hard, heavy, cumbersome boot at first, as my prosthetist made adjustments to the fit of the socket and the alignment of the carbon fiber foot. Clutching the silver bars beside me stiffly, I ambled from one side of the room to the other.

"Grab a video, Scott!" I suggested. "I feel like a toddler again, taking my first steps." We broke out into the song, "Put One Foot in Front of the Other" from the old Rankin and Bass Christmas special we'd both grown up with as kids.

Walking was definitely less painful than on my cobbled-together flesh-and-blood right ankle. But even with my definitive prosthetic, it wasn't the same as regaining my pre-accident limb. I knew it would take time to get used to.

This new normal meant new limitations. Everything took more time. Expectations for what I was able to do needed to be reexamined, again. And again. Picking out outfits was a chore, as my footwear was pretty limited (the shoes make the outfit!), and skinny jeans and leggings did not fit well over the knee of my prosthetic socket. If I needed to switch shoes, I often had to adjust the pitch of the heel height of my prosthetic foot and walk around the house, testing out each change of footwear. As I'd explained to each doctor during my amputation consultations, because my right sacroiliac joint was fused, it was very important that my leg length was equal, as walking any distance with a discrepancy in leg length would create inflammation in my lower back, and I would be in pain.

I grew frustrated that life was so dang unpredictable. Pain was unpredictable. Kai was unpredictable. My mood and my patience were unpredictable, and so were Scott's. Sometimes I felt resentful. Before my accident, our family was used to being active and on-the-go, often changing plans at a moment's notice. Scott's and my personalities had always been upbeat, defined by good-natured banter, wry wit, and humor.

Now that my life was filled with so much struggle, I felt robbed of the keen sense of joy that had once come so easily. It was hard to be the same person in our relationship when I felt hampered by my body in so many ways, while the ever-present responsibilities of parenting mounted. There were many times when I felt pressured by Scott to rally, to be the wife and mom I was before this huge life change, but it just wasn't possible. Trying harder and moving faster often meant wearing myself out. As I tuned into the new rhythms and patterns of my body, my innate tendency to give and give of myself to my husband and family needed to be corralled in favor of self-care. Scott's failure to understand this dynamic led to frequent arguments and a lot of tears. We all wanted to get back to the normal we had known—including me. But the harder I tried, the more depressed I became. I knew that there was no way Scott could put himself in my shoes to experience my reality, yet I longed for him to understand.

With an accident like this, with a limb amputation, there was no quick "getting over it." There was no swift "moving on." Even though the prior hurdles had been surmounted, I remained stuck in waiting mode. Feelings of stagnation loomed over me, punctuated by frequent annoyances and occasional bright spots.

But as was my known pattern, I persisted in trying to keep hope alive. Digging deep from within my inner emotional reserves, I continued to find reminders of my badassery. My strong constitution—a natural athleticism, mind-body awareness, and dogged determination—served as a good rudder in navigating the craft of this new post-accident life. *You have been through so much already and have come out the other side*, I told myself. *Setbacks are to be expected. Hang on.* I knew this would be tough for a little while longer, but we would get through it.

I continued reaching out to my new amputee friends, who provided a constant source of encouragement. About six weeks after my amputation, when my surgical site healed and I received the thumbs up to exercise, I made my way to the YMCA where I received a hearty "Welcome back!"

Swimming became my go-to activity, since it was non-weight-bearing and the buoyancy was a welcome reprieve from relying on my intact left leg. Every time I rolled onto the pool deck on my knee scooter, I had to squelch the automatic tendency to grab a kickboard. With my right foot missing, I now kicked in circles. Getting the hang of this new life would take some time. Some change is permanent. I would be footloose, but never truly fancy-free.

PHANTOM PAIN AND BURIED PAST

Lots of people in the limb loss community suffer with phantom pain. Once a limb is severed, the messages between the severed nerve endings and the brain continue to fire as if the limb still existed. It is as if the brain registers something is wrong and sends out an alarm system to get your attention. "Hey! Don't forget about me down here! Wait, what? Oh, never mind. I'm not here anymore."

For several months after my amputation, I continued to feel little zaps shooting into my non-existent foot and fleeting cramps in my absent toes. From all I had learned, I knew these phantom pains would be temporary, but they were still frustrating. I often felt a hot searing pinch where my pinky toe had been. At other times, it felt like someone took a vice-grip and bore down on the end of my big toenail for a few seconds.

Cerebrally, phantom pain does not make sense. How can your toe hurt when it's no longer there? Doctors employ specialized therapies designed to retrain the brain in an attempt to help the amputee relieve their phantom pain, yet often the pain persists. Those neuropathways are stubborn little buggers. They know something is wrong and they just can't get over it.

It's tempting to think it is easy to just retrain the brain. While my phantom pain eventually went away, for some folks it can be permanent and debilitating—especially for those who lose their limb abruptly through trauma such as a car accident or a bombing. I knew countless amputees whose phantom pain couldn't be trained away. They became frustrated and depressed by the pain haunting them.

In a similar fashion, I had read countless books about adoption trauma, and I could not help wonder if the same general principle applied regarding the emotional and physical loss of a birth mother. In my dealings with my son, I always wondered why he just couldn't connect with me. As hard as I tried, it was as if his biological wiring couldn't complete the circuit of connection.

From a logical standpoint, I knew we were giving him all he needed: love, nurturance, food and sustenance, affection. He had all his needs met and more. So why did his behavioral challenges persist? How could he continue to experience emotional pain? When I finally understood the connection between the brain's pathways and their tendency to search for what is known and familiar, I had a profound a-ha moment. My children were severed from their families of origin and their homeland. They'd been separated from these important parts of their lives before they were able to consciously understand what had happened—a concept written by Nancy N. Verrier called *The Primal Wound* (Verrier, 1993).

While it helped to acknowledge the reality of my children's losses, I still struggled to accept the fact that Kai could not love me back in the way I wanted him to. His involuntary response to keep pushing me away—through outright behaviors and daily interactions—felt maddening and depressing.

It wasn't until I realized his brain neuropathways had permanently been changed by his earliest maternal loss and the orphanage neglect that followed that I understood. The neuropathways which searched for familiar physical feelings had been severed for me, just as Kai's neuropathways for emotional bonding had been severed in infancy, not by surgery but by neglect, unpredictability, and abandonment. In accepting Kai's phantom emotional pain, parenting him became easier. In time, I gained compassion for Kai rather than frustration. I accepted that I might never experience a strong, emotional, loving bond with Kai, in the same way that the toes on my right foot would never feel cool blades of grass again. I would never wiggle the toes of, or be able to flex, my right foot. I accepted he might not be capable of loving me, and that was okay. I could love myself, and I loved him in the ways he would allow me to.

In the enormity of Kai's struggle, it was easy to forget Jade's experience in all of this. She had always presented well, as a happy-go-lucky kid. That changed in her teenage years, when hormones and surliness set in. She had insight about her triggers, but that didn't always make it easier. Intimacy, separation, and the tendency to want to "people please" were always problems for her. Her triggers stemmed from fears of abandonment and the threat of losing anyone—family, friends, boyfriends—left her seeing the world through the lens of fear rather than emotional mutuality. If she felt someone was mad at her, it was the end of the world. Being accepted, liked, and *wanted* were essential for her emotional wellbeing.

When Jade was little, she'd had nightmares. It seemed to take forever for her to go to sleep, so I often lay next to her on her bed and stroked her arm until she drifted off to dreamland. When all was quiet, I would pry my arm out from underneath her and tiptoe toward the door. Nine times out of ten, her eyes would spring open just as I was about to make my escape, and I had to tiptoe back to her bed once again. After a while, I discovered it was probably better to allow myself to doze off too, in order to avoid waking her in the earliest stages of her sleep.

Kai's separation trigger revolved around food, which continues to this day. He is unable to focus on his homework or his chores if his belly isn't full or if his next meal or snack is unpredictable. Food insecurity and hunger sends him into a dizzying tailspin. When Kai was younger, in-home Applied Behavioral Analysis therapists created a "food in sight" program for him, hoping to lessen or extinguish his tendency to obsess about food. They placed a treat on the table in front of him, directing him to focus for a period of time on the learning tasks at hand. If Kai touched the treat, asked about it, or tried to eat it before the end of the work time, they would give him a less appetizing snack later. If he succeeded in not obsessing, he was rewarded at the end of the session with whatever yummy goodness (usually a candy bar) was sitting on the table. The "food in sight" program lessened Kai's obsession with food—but did not extinguish it completely.

Whether dealing with issues of food insecurity, physical safety, or any perceived sense of emotional deprivation, Kai's hypervigilance never went away.

When Kai was in middle school, his physical education teacher wrote home. "Mr. and Mrs. Morgan, I just wanted you to be aware that we use heart monitors in our cardio unit. Kai is probably the only student I've ever seen whose heartrate is in the cardio zone throughout the entire class period!"

The gym teacher seemed to celebrate this aerobic feat. While I had intimate knowledge of Kai's operating in constant fight-or-flight mode, the teacher's email gave me reason to educate him on the reasons for Kai's constant hypervigilance and activity.

"We'll use that energy to our advantage," he responded when I explained.

Together with his guidance counselor, we devised a way for Kai to be the class helper (taking out trash, clearing tables) to redeem the energy he had in spades, since not all classes could be as active as gym. Teachers continued to comment that they wished they could bottle Kai's energy and drink it themselves. While maddening at times, we also found that tapping into his energy reserves could be beneficial.

As the years went on, Kai's combined interest in culinary arts and incredible surplus of energy landed him a job bussing tables at a prestigious Italian fusion restaurant in town. His co-workers loved him! Kai's infectious smile, dynamic energy, and ability to thrive while constantly on-the-go propelled him into the culinary community, which embraced him and all his quirks.

Kai began asking questions of the chef about what it would take to start a career in culinary skills. "How did you become a chef? Did you go to school? Do you like it?" He came home brimming, night after night, sharing how much he enjoyed his work.

"Guess what? Some customer gave me a $20 tip!"

I was proud and overjoyed. *I couldn't have made this happen,* I thought to myself. *Here is my kid—my once starving kid—thriving in a job in the restaurant industry, at the age of 15.* Seeing my son happy made *me* happy. I began to worry less about his future, and mine.

I could not wish his trauma away, or mine. But we could live into our futures with intention. And the healing would continue to happen, over time.

UPSIDE AND DOWNSIDE

I never regretted the decision to amputate my leg. In the same way the field of thanatology (the scientific study of death) calls the prolonged grieving experience prior to death from a terminal illness "anticipatory grief," I had experienced anticipatory loss from the moment I truly acknowledged that my ankle wasn't fixable. Like any terminal disease process (and the doctors who try to fix everything), accepting when you've reached the point of no return is crucial. People grieve and deal with this reality in different ways.

Of course, there were still aspects of post-amputation life that felt like a loss. While I had never been one to enjoy wearing heels, when I did my legs were the bomb. I had inherited both of my parents' well-muscled leg genetics: long, lean, shapely, and defined. Even though Scott is quite a bit shorter than I am, he often begged me to wear heels when we went out, saying, "You've got great legs. Flaunt 'em!" Like Dudley Moore and Susan Anton in the '80s, we gained some comedic mileage from the differences in our height when I wore heels. I relished feeling statuesque and sexy.

While manufacturers make prosthetic feet that give the option of an adjustable heel height, the mechanics of these limbs sacrifice bounce and what's called "energy return." As someone who prizes the ability to be quick on her feet and as active as possible, this type of foot was less desirable than some of the other prosthetic feet on the market. Insurance only covers one prosthetic foot every three years, so I sacrificed fashion for function and opted for a bouncier, high-level activity, carbon fiber foot. I still longed for the feeling of donning an airy, delicate summer dress and strapping on a pair of three-inch heels. That's one of the things I lost as a result of the amputation. Flats just don't complete the outfit or leave me feeling elegant and attractive in the same way. The prosthetic leg served as a clunky, heavy, and humbling reminder that life was much less carefree than it used to be. I couldn't look as chic and sexy I used to.

My pride in survivorship was mixed with sadness and loss, and, as in all things, I had to adapt. I searched for new and different ways to feel sexy again through experimentation with different hair and clothing styles. Flirtatious humor continued to be a cornerstone of our marriage and we defined a new sense of sexy, in a similar way that older couples embrace the quirkiness of aging with bodies that change over time. I tried hard to embrace this new normal. It was humbling.

Going to the beach with a prosthetic device can be a pain. With all my scars and aging body, I didn't feel comfortable wearing a bikini. I could no longer wear flip-flops with my prosthetic foot. When it came to the beach, sensible swimwear, sunscreen, a stylish cover-up, and a good bottle of wine replaced any former ideals. Sand and salt water wreak havoc on prosthetics, gumming up the works with rust, grit, and corrosion, which often creates further logistical setbacks (insurance, additional prosthetic visits for trouble-shooting) when returning home to life off the beach. Fresh water is less problematic, but keeping the leg on in the aquatic environment can get tricky; sometimes it's just best to take the thing off altogether. When kayaking, canoeing, or whitewater rafting, I opted to remove my leg and tether it to the inside of the watercraft because it is less cumbersome. The hassle was worth it though; I was just glad to be active again.

Wearing a prosthetic leg is hot in the summer. As I approached middle age and the onslaught of hot flashes began, so did the profusive sweating during workouts. Jade and Kai would often wrinkle up their noses and recoil, uttering an *"Ew, gross!"* when I took off my prosthetic liner, held it upside down and poured the dripping sweat out into the sink. These two had seen their fair share of grossness with all my surgeries, so I knew this was minor.

Some of the drawbacks of life as an amputee are offset by the fun and humor. Halloween, for instance, is always entertaining. One year, our family decided to be a band of zombies for a haunted house. Scott enjoyed playing the role of a chainsaw killer and pretended to tie me up with duct tape as he sawed off my bloody rubber foot. Our little skit was realistic enough that one poor boy screamed and hugged his dad saying, "Oh my God! I think he really cut her foot off!" Years later, we threw a pirate-themed Halloween party and of course, I was Peg Leg Patty. Scott concocted a great peg leg from a chair spindle and screwed it into the bottom of my socket. Nothing beats an amputee Halloween costume!

Details are important in the prosthetic world, and so are tools. Just like it did when I forgot to clip the auto belay, one big brain fart can make a huge difference. Forgetting to bring an Allen wrench, Loctite adhesive, or appropriate sock ply can make all the difference in whether I will enjoy the day or be miserable. Once, when back at work, my foot came loose and jiggled at the end of my socket as I walked. I had left my prosthetic tool stash at home, so I had to call the maintenance department to borrow a 4-mm Allen wrench. That turned out to be a quick fix; I was lucky. I kept a well-equipped stash of foot/leg tools close at hand thereafter.

These ongoing annoyances became good life lessons, which I applied to myself as well as to my children. Planning for a day of walking around on a prosthetic is not that much different than planning to walk into the snow on a cold Wisconsin winter day. Thinking ahead to *What might I need?* is always a great life skill, and my children absorbed this lesson early on through our family's outdoor experiences. There was a silver lining: when Jade and Kai became teenagers, their teachers often said, "They are so good with helping the other students plan."

Kai had an uncanny knack for noticing sequencing of events (especially if someone forgot a step) and Jade surfaced as a reluctant leader-type to her classmates. She was the responsible kid all her friends looked up to; she was smart and made wise choices. I often wondered if the universe had used my situation to carve out these subtle discoveries for both me and my children. Quite possibly, she did.

Our children's growth took place in the universe's timeline—not mine. While I wrestled with learning to live in my new, changed existence, I also learned how to read the subtle messages life tried to teach me along the way. *Slow down. Think things through. Be present in the now.* These life learnings unfolded for Jade and Kai alongside my long journey in a way that unexpected blessings do; evolving out of a reluctant dance with life's circumstances. Like many parts of life, these lessons are rooted in the dark, shadowy caverns of exquisite pain and must meander their way upward—sprouting in their own time and place, unearthing new strength and deeper wisdom.

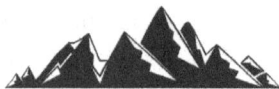

In August of 2014, the four of us vacationed in the Black Hills of South Dakota, planning to do a fair amount of hiking, climbing, and sightseeing. The bright, blue sky illuminated the gray granite and conglomerate rock as we toured the Needles of Sylvan Lake, Mount Rushmore, and Spearfish Canyon. Against the well-meaning advice from friends, we opted to travel during the Sturgis Motorcycle Rally, meaning we were joined by the distant rumbling of motorcycles as we camped beside a bubbling brook in Hill City. Jade and Kai waded into the water with their plastic shovels and sand toys and practiced panning for gold.

It was a memorable vacation, in that our kids were still the perfect ages (7 and 9) to engage in pretend play, and were also excited by every new experience. This included a 6.5-mile, 7,242-foot hike up Black Elk Peak, which we knew would be an arduous, all-day endeavor.

It was sunny, humid, and muggy—conditions made all the more suffocating by the dense foliage, which limited any natural breeze. Trekking poles helped me navigate my first long hike on a prosthetic leg. Periodically, I needed to stop along the way and take my leg off to empty the sweat from my prosthetic liner. By about the third mile in, the kids began bickering with each other and complaining about being tired.

"How much longer do we have to go?"

"Can we be done now?"

"Do we have to go the whole way? *Pleeese*, can't we stop and go back?"

Scott and I assured Jade and Kai that the view at the summit would be worth it.

"You guys, just wait! It will be so cool at the top," I told them. "We'll have candy and snacks at the summit in celebration of our efforts. You guys are doing great. It's going to be amazing. We'll take a picture!"

As the dirt trail meandered upward and the summit came into view, we noticed people taking pictures and selfies as they scrambled through the rocks at the base of the summit. Jade whimpered, smacking at her legs and stomping her feet. Each time we slowed down, she complained of getting eaten alive by mosquitoes, and she had huge red welts to show for it.

By the time we reached the summit, Jade was in full-on meltdown mode, crying and slapping her legs like some kind of crazy person. *What the heck?* I stopped behind her and noticed a small swarm of no-see-ums hovering around my shoulder. We were used to mosquitoes, but no-see-ums were different. I pulled out my bug-repellent, but it was already too late. Jade was miserable.

I pulled her close and kissed her on the forehead. "Let's just get a family picture at the top. The view is so pretty, we can't miss it."

Jade dried her tears and walked beside me as we clambered from the base of the summit to the peak, where there was a welcome, cool gust of wind; up here, the light, microscopic no-see-ums didn't stand a chance. We sat down to have a few snacks and a short reprieve from the bug drama before capturing our success on film. The gleaming, sapphire sky provided a scenic backdrop for a magnificent family photo shoot.

"Let's all raise our hands up in the air and say, 'Yay! We did it!'" I said.

Scott, Jade, and Kai did as instructed, and a friendly hiker took our celebratory summit shot. From the picture, one would never guess that our family's victory pose was momentarily hiding our daughter's snarl, or that on the hike down we were stuck with two exhausted, cantankerous children. Scott and I swore we would never do that again—with the kids anyway. While I was ecstatic to nab a great family summit photo, to this day, every time I see that picture, I recall the no-see-ums and my daughter's ugly meltdown. I think to myself, *This is life*.

Everyone has meltdowns from time to time, as well as aspects of our lives that don't appear in the celebratory photos we share with the world. Like the no-see-ums on our hike that plagued our bug-phobic daughter, the no-see-ums in our lives (the private, ugly things the rest of the world doesn't see) also plague us behind our daily facades. We try to capture the special moments even while we live in the thick mundanity of reality. We make progress but never achieve perfection. The journey is riddled with potholes, detours, and unforeseeable life circumstances beyond our control. We keep trudging on anyway.

STRENGTH TO LISTEN, COURAGE TO HEAR

I did a lot of soul searching regarding my career in the months and years following my life's extended detours. I could not return to social work: I had not kept up with the education and licensure requirements and knew returning to that type of field work in urban environments would not be a wise endeavor—for a number of reasons. My life had changed in so many ways in the fallout of parenting children from trauma and my accident.

I needed a new direction. The field of healthcare offered a exciting challenge. In a sense, I saw this change as an opportunity to embark on another stimulating, meaningful adventure.

Around the four-year anniversary of my accident, I noticed a deep appreciation for life's trials; tenderness of heart became unearthed within me, and I sought out a place to understand this change within myself. My background in theological studies paved the way into hospital chaplaincy, and I began the life-changing process of Clinical Pastoral Education (CPE). CPE is a method of learning based in self-reflection through learning to sit with others in their healthcare crises—without walking away from the pain.

We all deal with loss and at this point, I felt like an expert. I wanted to help other people in similar situations, understanding life's harshness and seeming unfairness. CPE training provided the opportunity to work through my losses alongside a trusted peer group and trained supervisor. It also gave me a comfort in going to hard emotional places and an ability to hold quiet space for patients and families when there were no easy answers. Death. Loss. Terminal illness. Change.

Sometime in my second unit of CPE, I developed a pressure sore on my tibial head—the bone on the lateral side of my leg, just under the knee. This is not uncommon for BKA amputees. Often, small changes in weight or activity level will affect how an amputee's residual limb fits in the prosthetic socket, creating friction and pressure under the prosthetic liner. I made an appointment to see my prosthetist in Orlando,

Florida, and he decided it was probably best to forgo use of my prosthetic leg until a new socket could be made. *Shit. Hobbled again.* While
I had suffered worse setbacks, I still felt defeated and frustrated. I had
just gotten into the mindset of living my life like any average person,
and yet here I was. Crippled. Beholden to my body's own timeline of
healing, limb changes that could happen at any time due to activity and
lifestyle changes, and the schedule of my prosthetist.

I called and left a message to Chuck, my CPE supervisor, sharing
the unfortunate news that I had to be out of my leg for the remainder
of the week, and that I likely couldn't visit patients.

"How can I help make it easier for you to get here?" he asked. "Can
I talk with security to have the hospital provide a complimentary valet?
Do you have crutches or do you need a wheelchair?"

Shoot. I surmised he'd have let me off the hook and grant me a sick
day, even though I wasn't exactly sick. I had expected to be hobbling
around while my leg healed in the eight weeks immediately after my
amputation, not now! In my mind I was whole again, accustomed to
having my prosthetic leg be part of me. It felt like a blow to be sans
leg, now that I was accustomed to having my prosthetic leg be part of
who I was, even though I knew the circumstances were only temporary.
Heading out without my leg wasn't in my game plan anymore. Every
time I thought I'd moved on, there I was again.

"Um, I dunno, Chuck," I hemmed. "I hadn't thought about coming
in without my leg. It just seems weird. I guess I could. Let me know
what you find out and I'll plan to get there."

I wanted a pass. I wanted to stay home and avoid the feelings of awk-
wardness that came with going into work without my leg. But I knew
Chuck saw this as an opportunity to grow, to mine the feelings of vulnerability that came with the experience. Exploration of raw emotion and
embracing vulnerability is the essence of Clinical Pastoral Education.

Chuck scored me a valet pass, and the valet staff helped pull my
knee scooter out of the trunk of my Jeep. I felt embarrassed as I noticed

subtle glances of folks curious about why there was no foot hanging off the back of my knee scooter, and I wanted to hide. But I couldn't. I knew I needed to summon up my inner bravery once again. I would have to take things slower than usual in getting around and accept help from folks to open doors and carry things. Even though I knew everyone was very kind and understanding, I hated the feeling I inconvenienced people by asking for help.

Fortunately, I did not need to visit patients in the morning because we had our clinical pastoral education group at that time. We students discussed our insights about ourselves, our patients, and our resistance to going into dark and difficult emotional places. Following group, I had my bi-weekly meeting with Chuck to talk about how things were going.

"Hmmm. I'm not so sure," I said, somewhat sheepishly. "I'm having a hard time thinking of rolling down the hallways without my leg. I'm feeling an avoidance to seeing patients and staff because I don't want the 'obvious' to be seen. I'm afraid I will become the focus of concern, not the patient."

Chuck expressed his understanding and validated my concerns, wondering aloud if there might be any clinical nuggets of vulnerability he might mine from our group discussions. "Is there anything else you might be feeling?" He asked.

I paused. Tears welled up in my eyes. "Well, yes," I admitted. "I guess I'm feeling embarrassed and kind of ashamed."

"Ashamed? Interesting. Why do you think you are feeling ashamed? I don't want to say it surprises me to hear you say that, but I guess it does."

I paused, looking out the open window. Orange and yellow leaves from the oak tree across the street clung to their branches as the autumn breeze gently shook them up and down. Some succeeded in resisting while others let go and drifted off into the wind.

"It's not that I'm not proud as hell that I've come this far," I replied, Chuck nodding his head in understanding. "Wearing my leg,

I feel whole. Without it, I feel vulnerable. I know that this isn't a bad thing, and it's something I share with patients—the vulnerability thing. But I think there's more."

Chuck smiled, fingers pursed together as he awaited my continued response.

"I think—no, I *know* that my deep sense of shame, here in the hospital environment, stems from my feeling like a rolling, legless poster child for medicine's failures. Like somehow, my worthiness came from my ability to show just how successful I could be at healing, and that didn't happen with my leg. Healing the medical way didn't pan out, so I chose to close the deal and move on."

"I see how you could feel that way," Chuck said, citing examples of visits he'd had with patients where they'd expressed feelings of disappointment for letting down their doctors or medical team. We swapped stories of instances where patients decided to forego grueling end-stage cancer treatments in favor of hospice, where they could spend quality time with their loved ones in "non-patient" mode for their last days. He also told me about his own experience of living with a chronic condition, where hospitalizations could arise out of the blue, without regard to his agenda or plan of action.

"Don't get me wrong. I know people stare," I continued. "They see me rolling through the hallways and see I'm missing part of my leg and my foot. I don't want pity. I don't want the attention. I just want to do my thing. It's different when I'm wearing a prosthetic because I feel badass. Rolling around without my leg, I feel pathetic. I don't like being a symbol of vulnerability in an establishment that prides itself on medical successes. *I didn't fail. Medicine didn't fail.* Our bodies will all fall apart someday, regardless of the advances in medicine and technology."

Chuck nodded again, leaning forward with his elbows on the table. "This is what makes you a good chaplain: your ability to *feel with*—to have compassion for others who also suffer and have similar feelings as you do. Those are great kernels of wisdom. Well done."

I did not get a pass from doing patient visits that day. Instead, I got a lesson in learning to accept myself as I was, to feel a deeper sense of belonging in this immense sea of flawed humanity. I also was able to explore the deeper emotions involved in the shared human understanding of physical, spiritual, and emotional struggle. As I fielded questions about why I was out of my leg, people appreciated my honesty and candor about living with an unpredictable ailment, not unlike those of the patients I served. Several staff shared that they respected me in my role, along with the fact I came in and kept keeping on. My colleagues shared, "You're a great role model for our patients and staff."

Sometimes, we don't get to choose how we influence people. To be able to offer true understanding and compassion to my patients, I knew I needed to accept my own vulnerability with loving kindness. It had to become a *practice*.

I may not have been able to stand on my own two feet on that particular day, but I was able to stand in my story, embrace my vulnerability, and own it as a catalyst for embracing self-compassion and shared connection. My prosthetic leg was eventually ready to come back to me. Life carried on.

My role as an interfaith hospital chaplain proved to be a meaningful and interesting one, filled with deep, affirming, and momentous interactions. At times, I felt oddly like a mole—sneaking around behind the realities of medicine; at the bedside of patients, capturing the raw, profound stories that would otherwise have gone unspoken. Like a heavy blanket, these patients' stories, faces, and lives envelop my heart. I was overwhelmed with an intense longing for resolution—yet often, solutions are complicated and elusive. While their treasured stories remain with me, I often leave patients' rooms with more questions than answers. Questions about healthcare decisions. Questions about reasons for treatments and futures that are uncertain. I ponder how life can irreversibly change in a heartbeat, and then just go on again. I curse the ebb and flow of personal power and powerlessness, both in myself and my patients. Here is where I have compassion for doctors and healers of all kinds. In healthcare, the unrelenting reminder of life's transiency is ever present, like the flow of water over a footprint on the beach. Now is all we have.

LENSES OF TRAUMA

After my release from OU Hospital following my amputation, Scott and I went into downtown Oklahoma City to order a sausage and mushroom pizza. I was hungry for a slice of normalcy and longed to get some fresh air while we were further south and could enjoy the warmer weather before heading home.

After dinner, Scott wheeled me down the street to visit the site of the Oklahoma City bombing. The government had constructed a memorial giving a history of what had happened, the names and memorial stones of the 168 people killed, and a little bit about the man, Timothy McVeigh, who had planned and carried out the bombing in 1995. I remembered McVeigh had been executed in 2001 (just a few months after the memorial opened) and that his last words were taken from the British poet, William Ernest Henley: "I am the master of my fate: I am the captain of my soul." *Odd*, I thought, *to utter such remorseless words right before a death by lethal injection.* I read that McVeigh harbored intense anger and resentment after his mother left the family when he was ten years old and that he became increasingly quiet and bullied in school. This had led to a preoccupation with violence and firearms in his later years.

As we wheeled into a large grassy clearing, I noticed a beautiful, tall American elm tree standing alone, its large lush leaves blowing in the breeze. This tree had been named the "Survivor Tree," as it withstood the huge blast, which killed and injured so many people and destroyed many of the buildings in the general area. The tree continues to thrive after all these years, a symbol of strength and resilience despite the death and destruction that surrounded it, and it serves as an iconic symbol of hope to all who visit.

Scott pushed my wheelchair up the bumpy, brick path to the base of the tree and sat on the ground next to me. I took a deep breath in and looked up.

"Hey look!" I pointed to a branch that had been cut, only to see a new sprig of green leaves defiantly protruding from the severed area once again. "What poignant symbolism after an amputation. Growth continues even after loss." I snapped a photo, which spoke to my heart, and thought aloud about the trauma suffered by so many, in that very area, almost two decades ago.

Scott said, "You are a survivor. Kai is a survivor. Our family are all survivors after dealing with such horrible adversity. It's fitting that we are sitting right here, right now, communing with all here who have suffered before." He reached over and give me a hug before wheeling me back to the car.

It occurred to me that I had become a student of trauma over the years, allowing the trauma to teach me things about life that I would never have otherwise known. Through this lens of trauma, McVeigh's final words began to make sense. Much of what we do—the habits we form, the patterns and the tendencies we have, the things we tell ourselves—is created out of a need to maintain a sense of safety in a world that can be unpredictable, scary, and dangerous. We crave mastery and control because we want to feel grounded when life is unstable and rocky.

The cumulative effect of parenting our son and living through my own trauma has given me a new and different lens for viewing the world. I liken it to an uncanny sixth sense, one that has been sharpened and honed over time. Kai's strong need for control, distrust of the world, and chronic hyperawareness of his environment all established their roots during his impoverished, early years. I know this. While frustrated with the domino effect of his trauma, I became oddly grateful for this new awareness because it has helped me understand the reasons why people do crazy and destructive things.

Looking back, I'm thankful we met Kai's needs, head-on and as early as we could, to avoid the potential of violence and pent-up anger in his later years (something many families face—especially when they don't understand Reactive Attachment Disorder and the importance of early intervention). Unresolved trauma can be an insidious disease with grave individual and systemic consequences. It is the crack in our collective armor that causes us to build up our arsenals of defenses to keep real and perceived threats at bay.

PULPITS AND PEDESTALS

I grew up in a small, closely knit Midwestern community of about 50,000 people where it felt like everyone knew everyone. I attended Catholic grade school and went to church with my family every Sunday. I felt secure and comfortable in this insulated community and have good memories of being taught by dedicated teachers, many of whom were religious sisters who devoted themselves to Catholic education and servant leadership.

It was the 1970s, just after Woodstock, the war in Vietnam, and the Second Vatican Council of the Catholic Church. I loved hearing stories where Jesus challenged the status quo and encouraged people to be compassionate to one another. I came to see Jesus as the sort of friend and role model who held me to a higher level of morality—engaging the world with a heightened set of principles that valued every person and living entity. Saints such as Dorothy Day, St. Francis of Assisi, and Mother Theresa held the torches of continued compassionate servant leadership amidst the changing difficult times, where the poor, the sick and the downtrodden were lifted up and promised hope and new life.

I attended camps through the archdiocese and later became a camp counselor. I taught confirmation classes and volunteered at the local meal programs. I had amazing role models and teachers along the way who, starting in my earliest years, instilled in me the value of helping others. It was not a huge leap, then, when the archdiocese offered me a scholarship in 1993 to obtain a Master's degree in Religious Studies. To me, the opportunity felt like a natural progression to obtain an advanced degree in a subject that had been influential in my upbringing. I welcomed the chance to make a difference in the world and to put my faith into action, working as a Director of Youth Ministry at a suburban Midwestern Catholic church.

During my first semester of graduate school, I learned that the parish priest, who spent thirteen years leading our congregation, had been accused and convicted of molesting a large number of students, some of them my close classmates.

"Father Bill? The man who heard my confessions year after year?" Aghast, I wanted to close off my brain to this knowledge, but I couldn't. I felt a sense of shock and disbelief. I could not understand how such a trusted leader—someone we called "Father"—could do such a horrible thing. My prayers to Jesus, my imaginary brother, went something like: *Hey dude. What the heck? I don't get this, do you? If you had a grave, you'd be turning over in it right now. You've gotta be pissed as hell.*

I'd always known Father Bill wasn't perfect. I recalled the countless times when I sensed something was off during Mass. Everyone knew Fr. Bill was an alcoholic by his stumbling around and slurred speech, yet the entire church community brushed the issue under the carpet, year after year. I remember asking why only the boys were allowed to go on camping trips with Fr. Bill, since I also loved camping and craved adventure.

"That's just the way it is," my teachers and my parents said. "You're not a boy. Only boys are invited." My classmates and I were told not to ask questions; we accepted that this was just how it was.

Fr. Bill was eventually sentenced to a lengthy jail term and died while serving time. I heard a rumor that he did not show any feelings of remorse for what he had done, which I found unsettling, because I wanted to feel a sense of closure and redemption. Instead, I felt a combination of disgust, anger, and sadness for this man, who I imagined had many inner demons and traumas of his own that went unresolved. He just kicked them down the road. Rather than healing his wounds, he became a perpetrator.

A fair share of clients in my social work career also showed no remorse for the crimes they committed. During discussions of wrongdoing, I saw their eyes glaze over in the same way that I would later noticed my son's eyes going vacant when he was younger and caught doing something wrong. There is a certain brain/body disconnect that kicks in as a defense mechanism to shield them from internalizing blame or accepting responsibility.

Shortly after leaving my job in ministry, I learned that the priest I had worked under for three years was the vicar for the archdiocese that had placed Fr. Bill in my hometown parish after allegations of pedophilia were made in his previous parishes. I wondered, *How could a whole community not know what was happening? Was the denial that deep and strong?*

Institutions of faith are supposedly built upon the greatest aspects of human strength, compassion, and generosity, created by the deep human need for meaning and human connection. That is why when violations occur within a spiritual community, the damage is profound and far-reaching. For me, Catholicism began to feel like a dysfunctional family that I needed to part from. I needed to sort things out and regain my bearings.

Anytime we are deeply vulnerable, we open ourselves up to deep hurt if that vulnerability is exploited. This is true with children who trust teachers, family members, and caretakers. Parishioners who trust their religious leaders. Patients who trust their doctors. The idea that

"I trusted you and you hurt me" wounds at the core level. We then build up emotional walls to keep further hurt at bay. I had started constructing my wall many years ago.

Not long after all my surgeries and hospitalizations, I started to acknowledge how the resentment from my early Catholic upbringing—with its tendency to place priests and religious leaders on pedestals—percolated just under the surface. I noticed the same repressed feelings and inclination arise in me as I deferred power to the doctors in making important decisions about my medical care. The notion that you don't question those in positions of prestige or authority was pervasive. Blind faith almost squelched my own voice until I paid attention to my inner rumblings and saw what was happening. I was thankful to have found supportive people along the way—other survivors of trauma, my family and friends—who helped me hold onto my voice and express it in places where it needed to be heard. Ultimately, I knew I would have to forge my own path—dogmas be damned!

As my daughter became a teenager, I recognized the benefit of having done my own inner exploration. Working through the buried feelings of disempowerment and unresolved trauma from my past helped her learn to claim her inner voice and feel empowered as a growing young woman. Jade continued to be a champion for women's voices in her high school and began an online sticker business, creating decals with memes such as "The Future is Female."

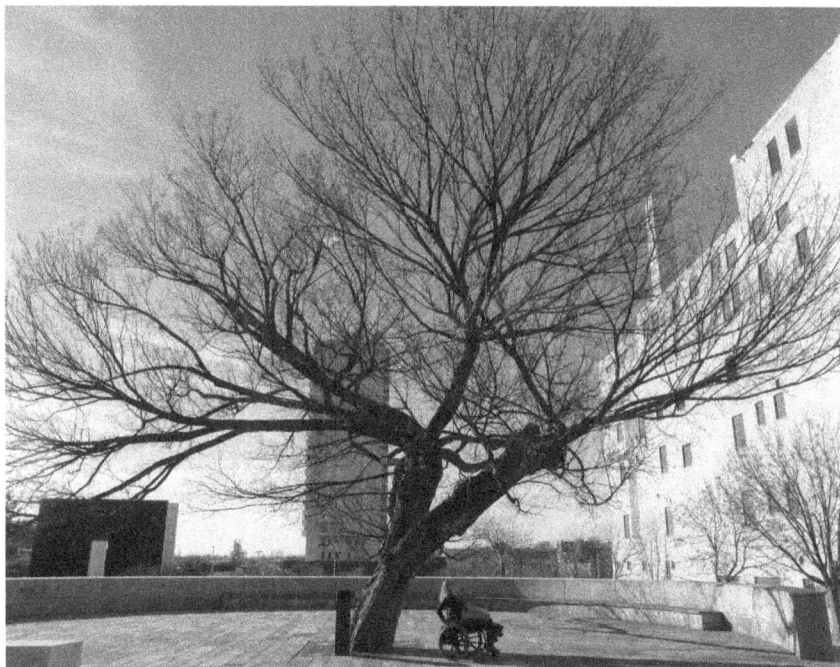

The Survivor Tree and me, Oklahoma City, 2013.

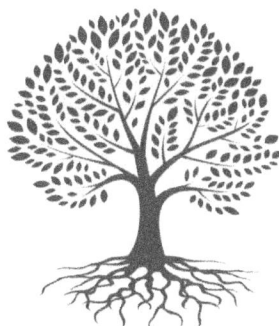

CHAPTER 7

COURAGE AND CONNECTION

Every September, I met the cycle of sending the kids back to school with a kind of strange, bittersweet nostalgia, an acknowledgment that yet another summer and another year had gone by. For all my grumbling and complaining about the work involved in raising both Jade and Kai, I love my little buggers and always missed them when they returned to school. With both Scott and the kids home every summer, I made sure to schedule memorable road trips to fun and exciting places, hoping to create experiences for us to take part in together every year. I was the bionic adventure mom, with no shortage of ideas for our family endeavors.

I wanted a normal life like everyone else; yet I didn't. I wanted life to be easier; yet my life was so stinkin' rich as it was. There was no way in hell I would give it up in favor of some picture-perfect family ideal. Life was deep and it was real.

A huge part of my identity resided in my ability to persevere despite my challenges and persist in being a role model of resiliency for my children. Even though I had lost count of the days where I wanted to quit and return to my former life, the deep-seated desire to be a mom and raise my children never left. Neither did my desire to make a difference in the world.

As I returned to career mode and began to work as a hospital chaplain, examples of life's sacred fleetingness continued to be magnified. Listening to the intimate stories of patients—their unmet desires, dashed hopes, and unfulfilled expectations—I began to feel a subtle twinge of panic. Life would continue to change in the years ahead. My kids would grow up. I would lose loved ones. Aging would cause my body to change in unwelcome ways and life would become more effortful. While hearing patient stories helped me become more grateful for my life and the people in it, these stories also heightened my feelings of responsibility to squeeze as much out of life as I could. The concept of time weighed upon me like ticking bomb.

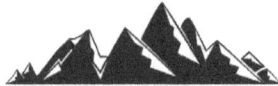

One busy Friday afternoon at the hospital, a woman named Barbara showed up on my consult list. There were a lot of patients to see before the weekend, so I did not have a chance to log into her chart to check the reason for the consult. I just knew I would be on her floor and decided to swing by to check in.

I gelled my hands with hand sanitizer, knocked on her door, and slowly peeked around the corner. "Good afternoon, Barbara. I'm Chris, one of the chaplains here. Is this a good time for a visit?"

A petite, older, African American woman wearing a powder blue nylon headscarf peered at me from her bed. Her small frame was well defined under her starched white hospital blankets.

"Oh, the chaplain." Barbara motioned with her fine-fingered hands for me to come in and sit down in the blue chair at the corner of the room. "I am so glad you're here. I have been waiting for someone to talk to, to try to process my unexpected news."

"Unexpected news?" I wondered what she had learned about her medical status and felt badly that I hadn't checked her chart. "Tell me more about what is going on." I sat back in the chair and got comfortable, because I had a feeling this would be a pretty involved visit.

Barbara looked up at me with an intense, caring, and sad expression. "They told me this morning that I have cancer—that I've had it for a while. They didn't catch it until now and it's too late." Barbara put her hands on both sides of her abdomen. "It's in my stomach, in my bowels—everywhere."

Barbara's eyes became glassy and brimmed with tears as she looked out the window and back at me again. "I didn't know this would be it. I had been having some stomach problems, but never thought it would be… cancer. I have been sitting here, wondering how I am going to tell my daughter. She lives in Indiana with her two boys." She paused again. "I have a meeting with hospice tomorrow and they want me to call her beforehand. I need to make that call but I am dreading it. I'm so glad you're here."

My heart broke for Barbara and for her family. "I'm so sorry, Barbara," I said. "I can't imagine how hard it must be to hear this news and to sit with it in anticipation of telling your daughter."

"I know… I need to call and tell her." Barbara continued to speak in a quieter tone. "I'm still trying to come to terms with all of this. I wasn't ready for the news. In my mind, this isn't happening. There is still a lot I want to accomplish." She paused again. "I'm not done yet."

Barbara went on to share that she was from Alabama and that she moved to the Midwest around 1970, just after the civil rights movement. She was instrumental in making inroads for human rights within the African American community in Milwaukee.

"I've always been one to strive for change, to encourage peace among people and listening amongst one another. For years, I have tried to promote hope and healing in the African American community at the government levels—housing problems and education in the city, anti-poverty initiatives, things like that. I have always had one project or another, even as I retired and became old." Barbara offered a shallow chuckle for a moment. "I'm 76, but the work is never done. There still is so much racism and injustice. I wanted to be a bridge, you know? A bridge to healing." She stopped for a moment as the tears slid down to her lap. "I *still* want to build those bridges."

There was a pause while Barbara cried for a few minutes. I could tell that thoughts were building up in her mind, and I remained silent to see if she would continue to tell me what she was thinking. "You know, it just, *just* occurred to me—" Barbara stopped and looked at me intently. "I think this is where I need to step back and say that my work is done here on this earth. Wow, it's hard to believe that I can finally stop working so hard."

I sighed while I tried to hold back my own tears. I knew I sat in the presence of a remarkable woman on the cusp of something profound and ground-shifting. Barbara was still so connected to her life's meaning and mission, yet learning that she needed to let go. The act of letting go was excruciating.

"How does that feel for you?" I asked, eager to hear her response.

She paused for a second before she answered. "I'm not sure yet. It's hard. You know, I've given so much of who I am to this purpose. I've seen a lot of things change for the better, but there is still a lot of healing to be done. I have seen wonderful and glorious things in my life—like Dr. King said, I have 'been to the mountaintop'—but there is so much left to do."

I continued to listen.

"But to answer your question," Barbara continued, "I guess I feel… a kind of relief." She looked out the window, then back at me, smiling.

"Yes, I believe I can finally stop all of my toiling now. My work here has finally come to an end." She exhaled, seeming to exude a deep sense of peace and serenity. "I never even imagined I would be saying this, but here I am, sitting in this room with you, and I can say that it feels like freedom. My prize is to be in God's glory."

I felt reverence and respect for Barbara in this sacred and intimate moment. My mind drifted for an instant and I wondered, *How would I react if I were given the news I was dying? That I had weeks or months to live while in the midst of living my life's mission—raising my children?* The thought was terrifying. Despite the obvious difficulty and no promise of its ending on the horizon, the idea of leaving my children and family horrified me. Even though my kids were teenagers now, they still needed me—and I needed them. *I have so much left to give. So much needs to be done.* I wanted to help them learn new things. To plan for their futures, witness their a-ha moments, and be present for their milestsones.

I knew that Barbara had harbored deep truth inside her and that she worked tirelessly until this very moment to speak and live that truth. I knew she embodied the stories of countless others who had endured generations of injustice, collective trauma, slavery, and systemic racism, and that every last cell in her body struggled and fought for her people. I could see in her eyes that she continued to care deeply about her mission and that she struggled to release her grasp from this intimate and personal life goal. Compassion exuded from within me as I looked with her upon the days ahead, knowing that letting go would be hard. I set aside my momentary thought tangent and focused back on our conversation.

"How does that feel for you?" I asked.

Barbara raised an eyebrow and wiped a tear. "Okay, I guess. I really have no choice." She sighed. "I would like to keep going, but I guess I have no choice. This is where my legacy will end, and I get to hand off the baton to someone else."

I began to feel choked up. I was sitting with an amazing, iconic woman and sharing in her grief. I continued to cherish every word spoken.

She continued. "I have done so, so much in my life. Been so many places, seen so many things. My life has been so, so full. *I am blessed.*"

"Tell me more, Barbara," I asked, as she seemed to cherish this ability to talk about her life without interruption. I had time to listen. I hung onto her every word.

"I grew up in Alabama," she started. "I walked with Dr. King during the civil rights era and knew all the people in his circle. He had a good sense of humor—that I remember."

"You knew Martin Luther King, Jr.?" I blurted. "Wow, to be a part of that slice in time must have been amazing!"

"Yes, it definitely was," Barbara agreed. "It was tough, hard work. You know how things were in the south during those times. The segregation, the lynchings. Oooo, those times were hard. But you know, we kept pushing ahead. Dr. King wouldn't back down and we made headway. It has always been, and continues to be, a work in progress."

I knew what she spoke of, living in Milwaukee, known to be the most racially segregated city in the nation (Spicuzza, Milwaukee Journal Sentinel, 2019). Fifteen years ago when I'd worked in the city, I had seen it begin to decay as businesses moved to the suburbs and left crumbling, abandoned buildings behind. The struggle of segregation, racism, and oppression of people of color was real, then and now.

"What brought you to Wisconsin?" I asked.

Barbara shared that her sister moved to Milwaukee and invited her to come up north, where the governor was more progressive and had an interest in social justice and improving race relations. With great pride, Barbara shared the human rights work she was able to accomplish in the city. We both acknowledged that we still had a long way to go, as Milwaukee *continues* to be the most segregated city in the United States.

"What are you most proud of?" I asked. "Looking back on your life, what do you feel best about?"

Barbara put her finger up to her lip and looked at me wryly. "Oh, there are a lot of things. But I think I am most proud of this one thing: when Barack Obama was inaugurated, I knew that this would be a historic moment. I knew without a doubt that I needed to take my grandson to the inauguration. And I not only took my grandson—I arranged a bus trip for his whole class to attend the swearing in ceremony." Barbara raised her hands up in the air. "Whoa, was that one glorious day. I'll never forget it."

"Wow, Barbara," I said. "What an amazing experience that must have been!"

After chatting a bit more, we returned to the pressing reality of Barbara's cancer. "When are you planning to call your daughter to tell her?" I asked.

She shook her head. "Today, probably after you leave. I am truly dreading this phone call." I offered to stay with her if she wanted, but she declined, saying that it would be a very difficult thing to do, and she wanted to have some space to let the emotions surface. "I could sure use a prayer though, if you would like to pray with me."

"Absolutely." I knew that Barbara was Christian and might appreciate something from the New Testament Scripture. "Are you familiar with Matthew 25? I can't help but think of God reaching out to you right now and embracing you, leaning into your ear and saying, 'Well done, my good and faithful servant.'"

Barbara reached her bony fingers out and grabbed my hand hard. I squeezed back. By this time tears were streaming down both of our faces. I knew her toil. I knew her strength. I felt tremendous gratitude for this moment, to be with her in her anguish. I sensed a sigh of relief that her labor on this earth was now coming to a close. It had been a hard, rich life, not unlike my own.

I walked over to the side of her bed, and Barbara happened to notice my prosthetic leg sticking out from under my pant leg.

"Oh, I did not notice your leg! Do you mind if I ask what happened?"

I gave her the abbreviated version of my accident and amputation, not wanting to talk too much about myself. I wanted to keep the focus on her.

Barbara looked at me, nodded slowly and uttered: "You are no stranger to suffering then. You know pain. Thank you for being here with me today in mine."

I briefly took a mental note of her overall demeanor. In facing her own mortality, Barbara was saddened, but deeply satisfied with her life's work and connections. I didn't ask, but I had a feeling she would say she'd do it all over again, despite how hard it had been. For a moment, I felt the same about my own life. Despite how hard it was—and would continue to be for the foreseeable future—I wouldn't want to let it go. Like Barbara, I knew I made a difference in the world. I saved the life of a child, but I also decided to stay the course when things got ugly, messy, and painful.

There was a time in my life I avoided pain. I ran from it in favor of the next fun and exciting adventure or worked to devise some kind of workaround solution. Now, I sat with it. I sat with my own pain and with the exquisite pain of other human beings. Had my accident not happened, had I not "learned to fall," I would not have had the presence of spirit to be still with Barbara without trying to run away from her suffering or attempting to fix it. Acknowledging my powerlessness and sitting with pain is, and will always be, the hardest thing I do.

I gathered strength from Barbara's witness and felt validated in my perseverance in working through the fallout of my son's trauma. Life had tenderized us both in ways we had not asked for, yet we persisted.

Barbara entered hospice and died shortly after our visit. I will never forget her.

WE'VE COME SO FAR

On my prolonged trajectory of recovery, I was reminded of the words of Philip Simmons from his book, *Learning to Fall*:

> We have all suffered, and will suffer, our own falls. The fall from youthful ideals, the waning of physical strength, the failure of a cherished hope, the loss of our near and dear, the fall into injury or sickness, and late or soon, the fall to our certain ends. We have no choice but to fall, and little to say as to the time or the means. (Simmons 2002, 3).

I have come to understand that much of life exists in the realm of dwelling in the possibility of hope and change. Healing and growth find their way in their own place and time. We may or may not get to see the results in our lifetime, and that's okay.

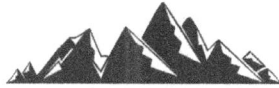

It was a cool March morning in 2018, damp and drizzly. Jade and Kai scrambled to get out the door on time for school, their backpacks waiting in the hallway. The previous month had been stained by a string of school shootings, and the whole country was on edge. Gun violence by and against young people had gotten out of control. Students at Jade's high school had planned a walkout in protest for this Wednesday.

I could tell Jade was grumpy as she stomped around the kitchen like an elephant and slammed her lunch box down on the counter, haphazardly stuffing her sandwich and napkin into it.

"What's wrong, honey?" I asked.

"Ugh. You know how we're doing this walkout thing in school? It's happening this afternoon and I'm going to miss part of my algebra class," she whined. "We have a test tomorrow and I'm not ready for it."

I knew that Jade's biggest source of anxiety was her schoolwork. A perfectionist to the nth degree, she tended to obsess about her grades nonstop, projecting a future of living on skid row if she failed to make all As. I continued to listen as she stomped around the kitchen.

"Ugh. I totally get this walkout thing with school shootings," she uttered. "It's not that I don't agree with it. I just want school to be about school and I want to learn."

I understood where she was coming from, but also knew that being a part of a student body making its voice heard would be an important life moment. I held my thoughts in and kissed her on the forehead as I assured her that she would have ample time in the evening to study if she needed to.

Kai bounded down the stairs carrying his library books. He was in middle school and had a vague understanding about the school shootings but did not dwell on them, which was a good thing. We tended to steer clear of this anxiety-producing subject, since both of our children were more inclined towards anxiety.

I hugged them both before they went out the door. "Good luck, Jade! Try hard today, Kai! Love you—see you after school!"

As I made my way back into the kitchen to pour myself a second cup of coffee, I thought about what had just taken place. *Was there more going on with Jade than I knew? Had the kids been more affected by the violence than I had realized?* My mind reverted back to December 2012. It was a year out from my accident, and I was recovering from another ankle surgery when a photo of the Sandy Hook Elementary School shooter, Adam Lanza, appeared on the news. I was aghast as I learned he had shot his mother in the head before traveling to the elementary school where he opened fire on 20 students and 6 staff prior to killing himself. The news report described Lanza as a fidgety and awkward young man, wracked by anxiety and problems with socialization. He was further described as a kid who displayed a lack of cause-and-effect thinking and struggled in school.

At the time, I felt a twinge of concern. My son's personality was a bit like this in his younger years. Awkward, fidgety, lacking cause-and-effect thinking. Suggestions of an autism diagnosis around age four. But Kai was almost six years old in 2012, and my family was different from the Lanzas in more ways than we were similar. We did not own guns, watch violent TV shows, or let the kids play violent video games. Our dedication and commitment to Kai's wellbeing persisted in soothing his simmering angst, and we saw signs of progress. He started reading. He loved building things with Legos. He began to show a keen interest in skateboarding.

I now sat at the dining room table with my coffee, six years later, considering all that had transpired in the years since the Sandy Hook shooting. I thought about Kai and felt grateful for all the progress he had made since 2012, thanks to the collaboration between his earliest therapists, teachers, and specialists and the hard work our family had put in from day one. I felt grateful as I looked back upon the teamwork and efforts, which I knew without a doubt had paid off big time. He was becoming stronger and kinder, with a tender heart for animals. He felt proud as he developed skills—at the skatepark and socially.

Kai was engaged during family time and excited about outdoor activities. "Hey Mom, wanna see me do an ollie?" he'd ask, proud to show off his newest skateboard trick.

"You bet!" *This is a kid who almost died*, I'd think to myself. *It's a miracle he's even talking and interacting—now he's rocking the skateboard skills.* I'd wonder, *What else does he have in store to surprise us with?*

I no longer feared for my son. I had hope for Kai and his future. He was actually turning out to be a pretty cool kid much of the time, when he wasn't irking his sister, dragging his heels, or draining his teachers by being the persistent class clown. In previous years, I knew each teacher couldn't wait to pass him off when the school year ended, but things changed as he approached high school. Teachers began to actually enjoy him in the classroom.

"While Kai struggles with attention," teachers would write home, "he is a fun and lively presence in class." One teacher shared that she loved his infectious smile.

My concerns changed from worry about his future to pondering what was typical middle school behavior and what wasn't. While my son still was very immature, he was, after all, a boy.

It began to dawn on me that my son's trauma (and our working it through) gave me a unique window into a world most people could not have known. A strong urge to write bubbled up to the surface. I pulled out my laptop and proceeded to bang out an article that I submitted to *HuffPost* (formerly *The Huffington Post*). "What Nobody Tells You About Parenting a Child With a History of Extreme Trauma" was published on April 14, 2018. A day later, I received a phone call from NBC asking if I would share my story on the *Today Show*. I felt dumbfounded. *Me? Really?* I needed some time to process what was happening.

Inviting a TV crew into your family's home is a huge conundrum to ponder. I wondered, *Would my kids be scarred for life from this? Would Kai's future be impacted? Would I live to regret this decision?*

I realized that the benefit of telling our story would help other struggling parents and far outweigh the risks involved in putting ourselves out there for the world to see. The issue of trauma-informed care was increasingly familiar in educational and other institutions, so the timing was optimal. My story, Kai's story, and our family's story could turn out to be part of another family's survival guide.

I was nervous as hell, but the segment turned out nicely. Our story was shared with integrity and paired with an author of a book about parenting burnout. The kids enjoyed seeing themselves and our family on national TV, and we watched a recording of it again together when I returned home from New York City.

I glanced over at Kai, now 12, who grinned from ear to ear as he watched the various images of himself on the TV screen. "What are you thinking, Kai?" I asked.

"I dunno." He responded. "I'm proud—I think?"

While our family had talked about this decision beforehand and agreed that it would be a good thing to do, I was a little worried that Kai would feel exposed or embarrassed, since the segment featured several pathetic orphanage photos where he was obviously malnourished.

"I had such a fat belly," Kai said, smiling and looking at Scott and me.

Jade piped in. "Kai, that's because you were starving! Your belly was swollen from starvation!"

Kai's smile turned into tears, as the magnitude of his earliest years began to hit him. "I'm sad," he said, crying.

"I know honey," I responded. "I'm so proud of you. You have come so far. *We* have come so far as a family. I'm proud of all of us."

I had hoped that sharing our story would help others, and it did. Countless other struggling parents reached out to me, thanking me for sharing my story. Many of them shared their relief in knowing that they were not alone in their efforts to raise children from troubled backgrounds. One woman mentioned that she had thoughts of suicide until she saw what I went through. She was so amazed that I persevered despite my accident and losing my leg. I was invited to do a couple of podcasts and speak to some organizations about developmental trauma and its impacts on the family system.

I was relieved to know that sharing my vulnerability and struggles created an opening for others to step out of the shadows of the trauma in their lives. In taking the risk, exposing all our scars and flaws, I invited discussion and connection. I was proud of being a survivor. I was proud of Kai. Revealing our story to the world was worth it.

COURAGE

The heart has always been linked to bravery. Even the word "courage" derives from the Latin word "cor," which means "heart." In his book, *Heart: A History*, Sandeep Jauhar writes:

> More than anything, the heart wants to beat; this purpose is built into its very structure. Heart cells grown in a petri dish start to contract spontaneously, seeking out other cells (through electrical connections called gap junctions) to synchronize in their rhythmic dance. In this sense, cardiac cells— and the organ they create—are social entities. (2018, 10)

It is well known in the world of cardiology that there is a strong link between the mind and the heart (American Heart Association, 2021). Psychological trauma and depression can cause heart problems, but human connection and nurture can mend them. I saw this in action while providing companionship to hospitalized patients in my chaplain role. I also felt it within myself as I pulled out of the quicksand of deep despair in my early days of parenting and recovering from my climbing accident.

As a recovering patient, I hated the isolation I felt when I left the hospital and no one other than my family got what I was going through. I felt like a burden, depressed and sad. Hopelessness and discouragement also wormed their way into the early days of my parenting. I felt alone, unsure, and terrified of the future. I needed to turn my worry to projects and goals as a way to process what was happening—to give it some purpose and meaning.

My experience as a social worker gave me the know-how to create programs during my healing phase to help people connect with others with similar experiences. I learned that the American Trauma Society website helped survivors of physical trauma and their families locate hospital support programs, so I met with the trauma department staff to help start a trauma peer support program at our own hospital. Within the year, four peer mentors were trained to begin meeting with newly injured patients on the trauma floor. The staff looked forward to our weekly visits for the hope and encouragement we gave to patients who desperately sought reassurance and support. We felt rewarded for giving back and offering support, since all of us had gone through a similar mental and emotional head game.

I also knew that I wanted to bridge the physical and mental aspects of recovery. I yearned to return to climbing again and I had a knack for creating programs to address unmet needs. I knew it would take some time and adjustment to figure out how to climb as a below-knee amputee, so I reached out to other amputees in the adaptive climbing world, did some research, and began to lay the groundwork to start the first adaptive climbing program in the Midwest.

After forming a volunteer committee at our gym, I connected with an organization called Adaptive Adventures, who would provide training and guidance. Dedicated volunteers and energetic occupational and physical therapy students from Marquette University embraced the program and helped it to grow wings. In time, people in the area with all kinds of disabilities—veterans with PTSD, children with vision impairments, adult survivors of stroke, folks with amputations and traumatic brain injuries—embraced rock climbing. The climbing community was accepting, and the program began to grow.

I enjoyed hearing the stories of people who, like me, had endured hardships and persevered. I craved these connections and cherished them. I drew strength and inspiration from watching folks summon the courage to climb up a 40-foot climbing wall—some with much more severe impairment than I had, like Pete.

Pete was a 70-year-old Vietnam veteran who lost the use of his legs after suffering the effects of Agent Orange. Pete spoke with a quiet voice but had huge, muscular arms, which earned him the nickname

"The Beast" in our adaptive climbing community. He had a wry sense of humor and a keen understanding of my son. I gathered that Pete was probably a little stinker himself when he was a kid, which was why he had the ability to laser in on Kai's subtle shenanigans. It was cute to see them hang together and to watch Pete give Kai driving lessons in his electric powered wheelchair.

One busy Wednesday evening at the gym, Pete was determined to climb the wall with green hand holds on the slab at the front of the gym. The route would be tough for someone without the use of their legs. Helpers were needed to keep Pete from swinging from side to side. The helpers were tied into ropes held by people belaying from the ground. I watched as Pete sweated his way up the wall, grabbing hold after hold with his muscular arms. His immobile, lifeless legs needed knee pads to prevent injury as he climbed upward, refusing to give up. As he neared the top, the entire climbing gym broke out into a loud roar of whooping applause. I looked at Scott. We both had tears in our eyes. We both felt proud of Pete, the Beast. Everyone who stopped to watch him expressed that they felt encouraged and inspired, in awe of his inner strength and fortitude. As Pete lowered to the ground and I approached to give him a high five, his smile was priceless.

"Awesome job, Pete. How did it feel?" I asked.

"Amazing," Pete replied. "I feel like a million bucks!"

Pete grew to be a sort of figurehead in the world of adaptive sports and athletics. His camaraderie was always welcomed and respected, and he later earned his belay certification, meaning he could help belay other climbers. It occurred to me one day, while I watched Pete belay another climber, that it feels great to lift people up (both literally and figuratively). It's empowering, satisfying, and meaningful. The gift of community and connection is priceless.

These days, support programs in healthcare are not well funded. They aren't revenue-producing, tend to be under-staffed, and often end up on the budget chopping block. Over the years, I've watched healthcare became more corporate and less connected to the patient experience. At their bedsides and afterward, I listened to countless stories from patients who felt increasingly alone in their pain. Sometimes, patients felt blamed for their maladies, which led to feelings of guilt and shame. Patient satisfaction ratings began to drop, and I knew why. Deep anger and resentment began to build up within me, because I knew that a huge aspect of folks' healthcare struggles originated from these feelings of intense isolation. As a desperate mom and suffering trauma patient, I knew these feelings well. I was lucky: I had the inner awareness, a supportive community, and the resources to help cope.

As stubborn and tenacious as I knew I could be, I started to realize that I could continue to spin my wheels advocating for these (non-revenue-producing) programs in the organizations I worked for, or I could shift my attention toward my family. I could continue to share my experiences with others and provide support where necessary, but my family—my lovelies—harnessed my lifeblood and filled my heart with great joy.

COMMITMENT

When Jade and Kai were 15 and 13, we decided to take a road trip out to Colorado and hike our first 14er as a family. A "14er" is defined as a mountain peak with an elevation of at least 14,000 feet above sea level. With 53 such peaks, Colorado has more than any other state. It is a memorable yet grueling full-body endeavor that requires an entire day's physical and emotional energy.

We approached Jade and Kai with the idea to gauge their interest, and we were surprised at their responses. "That sounds like a really cool experience. Let's do it!" Scott and I decided we would attempt to hike

Grays Peak, considered to be one of the easier 14ers in Colorado, with its well-marked path up to the summit and minimal technical difficulty. I brought up a few videos to show the kids of other folks making their way to the summit. They were psyched at the idea of working toward this cool accomplishment together.

We sat down and planned what to bring: lots of water, Tylenol for high altitude-induced headaches, plenty of snacks and food, layers of clothing, gloves, hats, good supportive hiking boots, headlamps, and trekking poles. I would need my typical stash of leg supplies—various sock ply sizes, an Allen wrench, Loctite, extra screws, and an additional leg (in case mine broke) for good measure. The kids agreed to get up between 3:30 and 4:00 a.m. so we could hit the trailhead no later than 5:30 a.m. Our goal was to reach the summit by 12:30 p.m., before typical afternoon storms would roll in.

As an amputee, I was the wild card. Even though I was six years into my amputee life, I had never hiked that distance at that high of an altitude. I did not know how to predict what might happen with my leg or my prosthesis. *Would I incur skin breakdown? Would I hold everyone up? Would it become painful as I got further out from the trailhead and too difficult to continue to the summit?* The kids and Scott provided reassurance. Kai even uttered, "Don't worry, Mom. You'll do just fine. If not, we can help you walk back."

We were successful in reaching the trailhead by 5:30. The beckoning sky was a deep royal blue, and the sun had just begun to peek over the top of the mountain range. Temps were in the high 40s as we headed up the gradual incline through the meadows, dotted with bright red, yellow, and purple wildflowers. We started out in good spirits and took occasional breaks when we needed to.

Kai grinned from ear to ear as he led our pack with his red and silver trekking poles. Jade pointed out the reddish-brown marmots squealing and playing off in the distance.

"I really hope we see some mountain goats!" she said.

"Me too!" Kai joined in. It made my heart happy to see my two knuckleheads embracing this family adventure as they trekked along the gravel trail.

Scott agreed to be our family pack mule, carrying additional water and my extra leg in his pack. We joked about our weird family: "How many families carry an extra body part with them? Who makes their husband carry their extra leg?"

Scott and I both worried a little about Kai. He had never been the kind of kid to put forth a lot of effort unless it was his idea to begin with. From toddlerhood on, he had a tendency to take the easy way out or give up altogether. His entire childhood, we had to remind ourselves that he'd been diagnosed with "failure to thrive" in his first two years of life. He needed to overcome a lot just to reach the level of his same-age peers.

We didn't worry about Jade; she was a different story. At a cleft lip/palate team appointment when she was three years old, our cranio-facial surgeon endearingly called her a "little bulldozer." Jade's strong constitution and iron-clad determination rendered her a little force to contend with even then. Hiking this 14er, we knew she'd do okay.

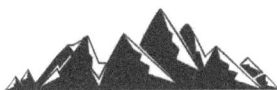

The air became thinner as we ascended the mountain.

"It's more work to keep hiking because it's getting harder to breathe," the kids remarked.

Kai's ear-to-ear smile began to recede and was replaced by abdominal cramping. My pack fit weird, causing my back and neck to ache. Scott developed an altitude-related headache.

"My knees and hips hurt," Jade complained.

We sat down on a pile of rocks as we reached the end of one of the switchbacks, about a thousand feet from the summit.

Kai was in tears. "My stomach hurts. I think I'm gonna throw up."

I stopped, removed my pack, and set it on the rocky ground beside me. My back couldn't handle the ache anymore either. My head pounded. So did Scott's.

"Maybe we should turn around and go back," I suggested. "Kai, are you going to be sick? Let's rest up a bit. Drink lots of water." Scott reached into his pack to grab a large Nalgene bottle of water and gave it to Kai.

Kai saw that the rest of us were committed. "Ugh. I want to keep going," he groaned.

The bottom of my nub was beginning to hurt, and I needed to make a few leg adjustments. My neck and back had started to throb in pain. I said to Scott, "I don't know if I can continue. This pack is killing my neck and my back. I don't know what to do."

Jade piped in. "We only have a little ways to go. I can see the summit right up the path."

A fresh-looking, young couple were making their way back down after reaching the summit. "You guys got this!" they said. "Right around the bend, you'll see a family of mountain goats!"

"Mountain goats?!" Jade exclaimed. "Mom, we have to keep going! I wanna see the mountain goats!"

Scott trudged over. "Chris, give me your pack. I'll carry it for you. We can't turn back now. We'll be at the summit before we know it."

I felt a combination of physical and emotional weariness with a healthy dose of guilt. "Aw man, Scott—I don't want you to suffer too." He had already started to complain of a hangover-like headache creeping in.

"No, Chris, just give me your pack. I'll be fine. We're going to summit this mountain, even if it kills us." Scott hoisted my backpack across his chest like a newborn in a front pack. The shoulder straps crossed over the other pack he wore on his back. We continued to climb, step after weary step, until we came to another clearing.

"Mom! The mountain goats!" Jade yelled.

"Where? Where?" Kai giggled, dropping his backpack and running to catch up with Jade. "Oh, they're so fluffy and cute. Look at them!"

Scott and I were both spent, heads pounding and dizzy. I was beyond sore. My nose throbbed with congestion. But seeing the kids ecstatic at the sight of a family of mountain goats imbued us both with the extra fuel we needed to keep forging ahead. The summit was now within our sight. We would make it.

Big, white, puffy clouds adorned the crystal-blue sky as robust winds welcomed us to the summit of Grays Peak. Scott dropped both packs and groaned, as he walked over to me and the kids with his arms open wide.

I began to sob. "Oh my God. We did it. This was so fucking hard, but we made it. Together."

Kai put his arm around my waist and watched my tears run down my cheeks. "Mom, you're getting all emotional."

"Yes, Kai," I replied. "I am. I'm so dang proud of you. I'm proud of Jade, too. I'm proud of all of us! This was so hard and you two did it. *WE did it.* Together!"

Jade meandered off to snap some photos of another cute mountain goat family lazing in the distance. Scott planted a long meaningful smooch on my lips, and we hung on each other while I buried my face into his shoulder. Pent-up emotion spilled out of me like rain into a gutter.

It was painful, treacherous, and grueling, yet it was also filled with deep beauty and joy—a strong difference from the previous family hike we'd completed years earlier at Black Elk Peak. The journey was long and unpredictable. It also held the promise of great visions and expansive, breathtaking views. We were tired and felt like quitting on multiple occasions, yet we rooted each other on and carried each other's burdens (okay, Scott carried my pack) when we felt we couldn't go on. We gained vast personal learnings, knowledge of the landscape and the changing temperament of the weather. We persevered, gained confidence, and built trust. The journey to the summit was not unlike our lives had been—painful, rich, profound—and we'd come too far to turn back now.

In the days that followed, Scott and I crashed hard. We wondered, *Would we do it again, knowing what we do now about how difficult the journey would be?* Jade complained of sore knees, but Kai continued to grin from ear to ear, basking in the glow this huge accomplishment. For a kid who had almost died so many years ago, he had finally come up from underwater and found his way to the top of the world.

Like giving birth, the pain and suffering is nearly forgotten when considering the payoff of a new beginning. A new life, rooted in possibility and growth.

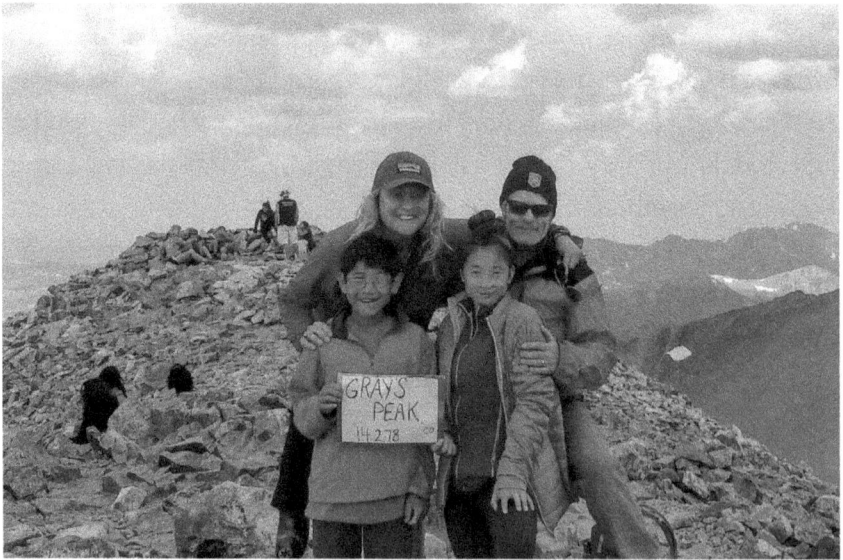

Summit of Gray's Peak (Colorado 14'er), Summer 2021.

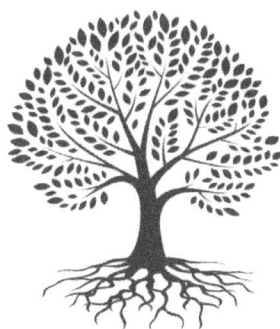

CHAPTER 8

LISTENING AND LIBERATION

> The word *LISTEN*
> contains the same letters
> as the word *SILENT.*

—ALFRED BRENDEL

In the late spring following my accident, I decided to teach the kids how to garden. Still on crutches for the foreseeable future, I was looking for meaningful, holistic opportunities for a seven-year-old Jade and five-year-old Kai to engage with me and the world around them. I couldn't run around, climb mountains, or create obstacle courses in the back yard the way I used to, so I figured I would find a different way to connect with the earth.

We invested in a collapsible, walk-in greenhouse from our local Big Lots store, just large enough for the kids to think of it as a kind of playhouse to grow things in. I bought packets of zucchini, tomato, spinach, kale, and bean seeds; potting mix; and multiple garden flats for us to plant them in. I purchased Jade and Kai each their own pair of mini-gardening gloves and individual little trowels for digging in the dirt and planting. Kai was excited to look for worms for our compost bin and learn about decomposition. Jade carefully placed the seeds into their containers and made sure to water them every day until the ground became ready for transplanting in June.

Morning after morning, the kids would scurry out the sliding backdoor to check if anything had begun to sprout. They were delighted when they finally saw green seedlings poking their heads out of the soil. When we were ready to transplant, the seedling containers were placed into our little red wagon and pulled over to the garden. I provided supervision, coaching, and direction as Jade dug into the ground and Kai handed over each ready-to-be-planted section. As the weather warmed, we watched in anticipation as things began to grow.

There were a lot of things about gardening I didn't know. I didn't understand that some plants did better with partial shade while others needed full sun for most of the day. I didn't realize that some seeds germinated more quickly at the start of the summer months, producing a prolific harvest before "bolting." I had no idea there was a planning process involved in maximizing garden space when certain plants completed their growing cycles. I just knew that I wanted to grow stuff, and I wanted to share this experience with the kids.

Everything takes time to learn, and gardening is no exception. We watched in disappointment as the tomatoes died because we planted in the corner of the backyard under the shade of the pine tree where they didn't get enough sun, while the lettuce we planted in the front of the sunny garden burned around the edges and bolted. After some time, I thought to myself, *You probably should have planned a little better—or at least asked someone knowledgeable about gardening.* I've never been very good at asking for help or advice. But the good thing about getting older and gaining perspective is that you realize what you suck at and what you need to work on.

For the most part, Jade and Kai enjoyed gardening when they were little. As they grew older—not so much. It was dirty and unpredictable, and it took a lot of effort. Gaining a prosthetic leg meant squatting down to ground level was out of the question, so we built a few raised garden beds. We did our research and tried to plan better for the growing season. Kai remained the compost king and became well acquainted with all things compostable. When his seventh grade class started a "green club," Kai was quick to sign up and take on responsibility as an organizer. Kai valued being a good environmental steward, something he shared with other kids.

I learned the benefit of companion planting, with wildflowers embedded alongside vegetables needing pollination. I moved my tomatoes into a sunny location and figured out how to rotate crops into my garden beds at the appropriate times of year. Spinach loved late spring and early fall. Peppers took a while to establish before proliferating in August. As hard as I tried to make my garden grow, I could only nurture the process along. I could provide the best possible conditions for my produce to thrive while nature made it happen. It wasn't much different from parenting.

When we moved to a different home closer into the city, I transplanted three bright, pink peonies, two bleeding heart plants, and two Asiatic lilies. There was something about hanging onto these heirloom plantings (especially the lilies) that spoke to me, and I didn't want to leave them behind. With the kids' help, we created a small garden along the front sidewalk of the new house, adding several hostas, grasses, and purple coneflower. Each season, we'd find something interesting to add, including a 12-inch meditating Buddha statue and a smiling copper sun. Sitting in my front office overlooking the garden, sometimes

I'd peer out and see passers-by smiling as they pointed at the various whimsical aspects of our garden, which grew and blossomed with each passing year.

"Wow, we sure get a lot of comments from the neighbors on our lush front garden!" Scott said to me one afternoon, beaming. "You and the kids sure did a good job getting that established all those years ago."

In more than one way, I'd think to myself. The toil and the digging, the planting, the nurture and the tending-to—these all come with delayed gratification, kind of like parenting.

Kai's early developmental neglect and malnutrition caused lags in learning and emotional and physical maturity. But like the garden, regular tending and nurturing produced growth. It took warmth, time, and patience through the turning of the seasons.

As Kai reached his adolescence, his physical development was aided by growth hormone stimulation therapy in the form of a daily injection—which he gave himself! Kai grew a whopping three inches within the first six months of his thirteenth year and gained an entire shoe size. While this didn't help his emotional maturity to catch up, it helped other people to treat him less like a rudderless, fledgling grade-schooler and more like the middle schooler that he was. The results were slow and steady, but they came in time.

As our kids grew tall alongside our garden, I started to realize that I could help by providing the right conditions for them to thrive—the warmth of nurturance, the showering of affection, and experiences of richness for learning—but that their growth would be determined by their own volition. I could do my best to finely tune my awareness to their inner stirrings and guide them like a master gardener, yet like any fertilization process—whether using chemicals, compost, or manure— the work and the waiting can really stink sometimes.

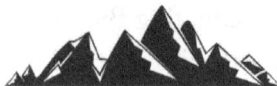

As a chaplain, every time I approach the door to a patient's room, I have a choice. I can knock, open it, and walk in, or I can turn around and walk away. Walking in and sitting down with people in pain means opening myself up to vulnerability and facing the deep, pressing issue of loss. Loss of life. Loss of control. Loss of hopes and dreams. It spins me back around to the lives of my children and their earliest years, hidden in the darkness and the shadows—with no sense of security.

While Jade had an occasional meltdown from time to time as a child, it wasn't until she became a teenager that the ghosts of her past would re-emerge. As Jade approached age 16, her previously happy-go-lucky, spunky personality began to turn a tad dark and surly. She spent long periods of time alone in her bedroom with her door closed, stopped going to fun social functions, and intensified her already laser-focused preoccupation with getting straight As. This intensity didn't calm down when she turned 17 either. I wondered why this sudden change had occurred. *Was this normal teenage development? Was it an adoption thing? Was she resentful towards us, after so many years of needing to be the "good kid" because she knew her little brother was a project that required so much work?*

Out of necessity, Scott had taken on a sort of case manager role with Kai over the years. On one hand, this arrangement worked out well because Scott wasn't a female and therefore Kai saw him as less of a threat than he did me. It took some time for me to let go and be okay with deferring to Dad. I knew that for Kai to succeed in the world, he would have to be able to trust someone, and Scott could be that non-threatening person. On the other hand, it seemed to cause a gendered rift in the family. While Kai was able to bond with and attach to him, Jade developed a seething, growing resentment toward Scott, and eventually so did I.

The first week of summer 2021, during break after the kids' freshman and junior years, Scott and I got into a huge, full-on verbal argument. What began with a discussion about finances and plans for the summer ended with my stomping out of the house and driving an hour away to spend a three-day weekend with my folks. Our home felt like a pressure cooker that I longed to escape, boiling with Jade's and my resentment toward Scott for being emotionally unavailable and Kai for consuming so much of his attention.

Scott was preoccupied and overwhelmed with financial concerns. Mounting medical and auto repair bills threatened to derail a family vacation that I had looked forward to for months and months, hoping to shake off all the stress we'd been under.

"We need this vacation!" I'd exclaimed to Scott, feeling the pressure of time pressing on as I knew Jade would soon be off to college the following year.

We had spent so many years growing a family and making memories. Despite all the hardship, I wanted to hold on for as long as I could to the family we had built and the experiences we'd enjoyed together. While I looked forward to seeing our daughter grow and spread her wings, I also felt a sense of dread as I thought about her leaving home. A family vacay felt like the best way to savor our last summer together and to override the difficult feelings that had begun to creep in.

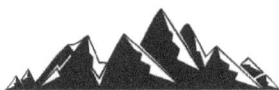

Despite the argument, I came home and we reconciled. We did in fact get to take a vacation: a spontaneous road trip out to Colorado, including a day trip to Boulder and a hike up the Flatirons. On the day of our hike, it was cloudy and drizzling, but we had all brought our waterproof hiking boots and rain gear. I hoped that a family hike would spark engaging conversation and fun banter as it had so often in years past, but this time the mood felt different. Jade had been moody, quiet, and distant, and I didn't know why.

The kids darted up the path before us. I grabbed my trekking poles, backpack, and water, and started walking up the dirt trail with Scott to catch up. I felt frustrated that I was much slower than the kids, needing frequent stops for prosthetic adjustments. "Can't the kids wait up for us?" I complained to Scott. "What's going on with Jade? Something's off. I've had enough of her surly attitude."

"Yeah, I've noticed it too," Scott replied. "I dunno, Chris, but I'm tired of always dealing with one thing or another with these kids."

"I know," I agreed. "It really bothers me that she seems to not care. I feel like she's shutting us out, and it hurts."

I asked Scott to hold my trekking poles as I texted Jade: "We can't see you. I have no idea where you guys are. Can't you wait up for us?"

Scott and I continued hoofing up the gradual incline of the dusty dirt path toward the first flatiron. We came to a series of stone steps that circled around a large oak tree and saw Jade and Kai perched on top a large granite boulder waiting for us to meet them. Jade looked down at her phone, rolled her eyes, and said nothing.

I couldn't take the tension any longer. "Jade, what is your fuckin' problem?! What's with the attitude?!"

She stamped her foot, slapped her thighs, and her face turned beet red. "*My* problem? Oh my *God*, Mom. You're so damned insensitive!" Hikers continued trekking past us, trying to ignore our mother–daughter spat, which was growing louder and uglier by the minute.

"Hold on young lady," I responded. "You're the one acting all entitled and pissy, like the world owes you or something. I don't know what's going on with you, but I'm tired of taking the brunt of your attitude."

"Ugggggh!" Jade began to stomp her feet, pacing back and forth before getting into my face. "You really don't get it, Mom, do you? *You left me! You fucking left me!*" Tears streamed down her flushed cheeks, and snot flew out of her nose. Like an angry, cornered bull, Jade continued.

"I'm pissed, Mom, I'm so pissed! Don't you know how much it hurt me when you just left?! You triggered all my abandonment issues, and I just can't get over it!"

My mind continued to spin. She was upset that I'd walked out after my fight with Scott. I felt guilty, but I also didn't. I'd needed a break from the stress of our family and my marital challenges. I had let Jade know what was going on, assuming that she was 17 and would be pre-occupied with her own life anyway. I had assumed she'd be fine—yet apparently she wasn't.

The argument on the side of the mountain continued to spiral, with Jade releasing her unbridled anger at Scott, Kai, and me. Other hikers and walkers quickly continued past us as we cussed and yelled at one another.

"I'm going back to the car!" Jade shouted.

"Oh, no you're not," I responded. "We're hiking to the top of the second flatiron, whether you want to or not."

"Ugggh! I hate you!" Jade continued. "You never fucking understand me. You think because you adopted me, I should just fit the mold of white people, but I don't!"

We returned to the path, making our way to the middle of the second flatiron. Jade was still in tears.

"Just give her some space," Scott encouraged. "You both need some time to cool off."

I knew our entire family suffered with some form of post-traumatic stress. Jade was in fight mode, I had been in flight form, and Scott's propensity was to freeze—either shutting off his brain with a distraction or crashing from emotional exhaustion in the form of a nap.

We were living our lives on autopilot, pretending not to see that Kai's trauma had impacted us all. But Jade's deep feelings of abandonment never went away either. Tears came to my eyes as I mourned for all of us and the losses we'd endured. The emotional pain bubbling up during this hike was underscored by a painful bottoming out in my prosthetic socket, made worse by the trek back down the path. *Man, I thought, I miss pain-free, hassle-free, and stress-free days.*

Slowly, we made our way back down the dirt trail, stopping at a clearing in the meadow at the base of the trail. Jade sat on the top of a large log bench and looked off into the distance. The rain had abated. A warm breeze swept softly over the meadow, blowing the strands of hair framing Jade's face. She was tired, and so was I.

"Come here, honey," I said, walking over and grabbing her shoulders to pull her in close. She buried her head into my arm and cried. Tears rolled down my cheeks and splashed onto the top of her dark ponytail. I brushed the hair from her face and kissed her forehead several times. "I'm so sorry, Jade. You know I'd never leave you. I love you so much. You're my daughter. I feel so bad that I've hurt you."

"I know. I'm sorry I yelled and swore at you," Jade said. "I get these big feelings, and they're so scary. The feelings just come over me—out of nowhere. Being different from you feels... isolating. Every time I look in the mirror and realize I'm Chinese and I don't look like you and Dad, I get triggered. I can't help it."

Scott leaned his elbows on the split rail fence, his face looking sad and preoccupied. Kai sat next to him, watching the hikers coming and going on the trail.

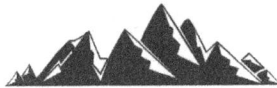

"You know I hate arguments," Scott said when Jade and I were done talking. "But I guess that's one that needed to happen."

I thought back to our family's beginning, when I wanted to close off my mind to my children's early traumas and losses. To conform their realities to my own wishes for the picture-perfect family, devoid of any challenges or difficulties. My kids have kept me honest and Scott has kept me grounded. I'm thankful that I held on tight for the ride, now that the aftershocks of our storms have subsided and the clouds have begun to part. I now bow to these struggles, grateful for what they have taught me. The journey continues, and I've learned to trust the universe in its humble, unpredictable unfolding.

I thought of models of resiliency I knew: my patients, like Barbara, other RAD parents, and other trauma survivors. We cannot run from our pain or our past. My children have taught me that suffering that's buried always finds its way to the surface. If the pressure is not eased or abated in time, we can spin out of control.

BLAME, SHAME, AND RESTORATION

Two months after my amputation, I was still without a prosthetic leg. Insurance denied (yes, denied) the claim, requiring my doctor to send a letter of resubmission to my insurance company. I was frustrated—no, incensed! *How* could an insurance company deny a person a leg to stand on? It's pretty customary for insurance companies to exploit reimbursement loopholes when dealing with durable medical equipment companies, who had limited lobbying power in Washington compared to that of the insurance giants. Unlike the pharmaceutical and insurance industries, the prosthetics industry did not have the capitalistic foothold (no pun intended) to create revenue, and practitioners were left scrambling for the pittance of reimbursement provided by competing insurers.

For a time, my heart sank into hopelessness and despair. *Would I ever walk again? Would I ever be over these enduring setbacks?* I took to the internet and reached out for support from other amputees who knew the struggle. Most were supportive; some were not. While my prosthetic leg was ultimately granted approval on the second go-around, I gained a lot of perspective in the process of reaching out and asking for help.

The implication that "you aren't trying hard enough" ran rampant. As I struggled to continue raising my children, one with special needs, as a newly disabled mom waiting for a leg, I could not believe the judgment I found on the social media limb-loss "support" pages. I read sentiments like "I found myself a job, so can you," and "Social Security Disability Income is for those who are lazy," and while not directed at me, they saddened me. Where was the compassion for others who were struggling? These harsh comments were far more common than I had ever anticipated they would be. While my family had financial challenges due to our the unexpected costs of life circumstances, I didn't dare share my experience for fear of judgment and disdain. I swallowed my despair and kept our struggles to myself. Another thing that disappointed me in this realm was seeing the failures of the non-profit industry. While there were great organizations out there, with missions to create community and encourage peer support, they scrambled for funds to continue their missions.

As my projected recovery turned out to be longer-term and more chronic in nature that the quick-fix I'd hoped for, I grew increasingly isolated. I began to see patterns of judgment on the Facebook pages that I followed which alluded to the concept of "strength" as an individual attribute. According to these posts, resilience had nothing to do with one's support system and everything to do with personal determination—something I knew was not even remotely accurate. Between raising my son and recovering from my accident, I'd learned that inner emotional fortitude was one thing, but it was nothing compared to the support of a village.

As my physical healing journey continued alongside my professional launch into the healthcare field, I worked hard not to internalize feelings of shame that I could not be the poster child of complete physical healing. I knew that the structures I found myself within were partially responsible for the chasm between the ideal and the reality. Parenting children with histories of trauma was much the same. We felt pressure to prove we had triumphed and prevailed. This was a far cry from the reality of our ongoing daily struggles, which truly never went away.

I attended trainings about suicide prevention and the opiate crisis in medicine. As a chaplain, I would continue to hear stories of patients feeling stuck and unheard. I knew these patients' struggles well and felt their pain deeply. The same achingly vulnerable questions pervaded:

"If I ask for help, will I be judged?"

"If I want relief from my pain, will I be labeled an addict?"

"If I share my feelings of despair, will I be locked up?"

In my adoption parenting circles, similar questions arose, surrounded by similar structures rooted in blame and shame.

"If I share what I'm going through, will I be labeled a bad parent? Will I be deemed as an unfit mom, or worse, will my children be taken away?"

While a great deal of foster and adoptive parents do deal with violence and child-to-parent abuse, I was thankful that never transpired for us. Motivational challenges and passive-aggression? Sure. But fear for my life, my safety, or the safety of my family? Never.

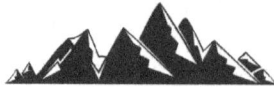

Healing is an ongoing process. Success and perfection are elusive pipe-dreams, in both medicine and parenting. Humans are, by our nature, always works in process. The need for each other and the need for understanding are as critical as the air we breathe.

I've learned that behaviors are messages. It took me a lot of time to realize with my son that his thwarting of my affection, his resistance to putting forth effort, and his subtle sabotage of self-progress were not personal slights against me. They were manifestations of deep, hidden wounds that will never go away. Kai embodies the issues that I continue to see in so many people who strive to be understood, just slightly more openly than some.

At times, it was incredibly hard to look beyond Kai's behaviors to see a wounded child, afraid of being once again rejected, judged, and abandoned. My heart aches for the adults who never had the chance to heal from their early childhood traumas. Where there was no nurturing "other" to provide comfort. No sense of safety or attempt at understanding. No resources available to work towards regaining some of what was lost. Many of these folks go on to "present well" and secure jobs with prestige or power, while resentment and anger continue to simmer just under the surface, and the illusion of "success" further hides their pain. Others do not fare as well and become plagued by their demons. Some end up in prison or rehab. Or a morgue.

The collective, angst-ridden cry to be seen and heard in our pain is a universal call to come together and to heal. It is what the Dalai Lama meant with his words "Compassion is the radicalism of our time." We are all hobbled in our own ways and trying to find our path back to connection.

THE BALM OF CALM

The word "compassion" comes from Latin roots: "pati," which means "to suffer," and the prefix "com-" means "with." To *suffer with*. To *feel with*, as Chuck said to me back in my CPE class. To have compassion, we need to know how to listen.

I have noticed that it can be hard to listen when I am preoccupied. In fact, as I sat down to write this book, I was met with countless examples in which I did not listen to my children or husband very well. While listening is important, so is laser-like focus. It is tempting for me to think, *If only I listened better*, or *If only I focused better*, then life would magically unfold in ways that are desirable and good. But it takes no time at all to realize that there is no "getting it right" in life. We are all doing our best with what we have.

It has taken a ground fall for me to gain some understandings. I have learned most of all from facing my own pain, from taking it by the hand and allowing it to show me my dark, rich, and tender places.

These tender places that hide in the shadows are where seeds of growth and connection are born. As Philip Simmons aptly shares in *Learning to Fall*:

> You see, we really are all in this together. Our journey takes us to suffering and sorrow, but there is a way through suffering to something like redemption, something like joy, to that larger version of ourselves that lives outside of time. (2000, 153)

Now that the kids are nearly grown, Scott and I will now often look at each other and comment that we don't need very much these days to feel fulfilled and happy. Like the boy perched on a stump at the end of *The Giving Tree*, we feel tired and proud, looking back on the painful, hard, rich, adventurous lives we've lived.

Yes, the tree had been ground down to a stump. So had my leg. We have all sacrificed a great deal in our lives and will continue feel the pangs of those losses as long as we walk the earth.

It's tempting to ask if we'd do it all again. I think that's an unfair question. It's impossible to know what life has in store. My kids didn't get to choose their fates, and neither did I.

We live, lose, and learn—and then wake up each day to begin again, hoping that we've learned something to grow from and build upon. Change can happen, sometimes slowly or painfully. Growth takes time. It's only when we know ourselves that we can begin to assert our needs.

The limitations of my body have asserted themselves more and more over the years as I've approached middle-age. Cold, damp, Midwestern winters are hard. My bones ache. I need to stay active and moving or I feel like the Tin Man in need of an oil can. Still, despite all these challenges, Scott and I joke that our relationship has stood the test of time.

"I love my wife with all my heart," Scott will profess. "All three quarters of her." My kids will joke that we're like the poster family from the Island of Misfit Toys, and it's true.

For one whose giving tendencies are deeply entrenched, focusing solely on myself was almost unheard of. It took falling, becoming shattered and broken, to force me to "take a break from normal living" and rethink everything. I had lived my life in full-on giving mode since forever, with little attention paid to my own important needs or the things that sustained my own tender wellbeing. I saw just how unsustainable it all had been.

It seems "falling" became synonymous with "letting go," releasing my grasp of control and desire to make a difference. I had to tend to the seed of my own inner growth and rebuild—which is easier said than done. In my reflections, I'm brought back to many of my fundamental theology classes, where I'm reminded that surrender is at the heart of all true spirituality. Faith is holding onto hope, letting go of control while grasping for greater purpose and meaning. We don't always get to understand the journey, and that's okay.

As I watch my children grow into stronger, more authentic versions of themselves, I am truly in awe of their strength, courage, and resilience. Jade has, in fact, started working in healthcare. Kai has his sights set on the culinary arts. Or maybe he'll go into another hands-on vocation—a far cry from what I feared long ago, as I sobbed on the bathroom floor of the neuropsychologist's office in Virginia. It's been tiring, hard work for sure, but I'm happy and I'm proud.

Scott and I just keep plugging and bumping along like we always have, chiding each other with regularity and keeping each other on our toes—which would be all five of mine. I've learned about falling and rising. About humility and hunger and longing. I think I'll always harbor a secret yearning for us all to understand one another. To put aside our defenses and see that we're all just trying our best to find connection and healing from the shards of our brokenness.

As Simmons so eloquently concludes in *Learning to Fall*:

> I've grown suspicious of perfection, seeking not a perfect life but a full one. I wouldn't go so far as to say that I'm *thankful* for my struggles, per-se. But I know that I'm able to appreciate the bright moments more intimately only because of the darkness that has surrounded them. (2000, 36)

Such is life. It's a delicate balance between giving and receiving, rising and falling, and cracking open over and over again into the bittersweet mystery of life's unfolding.

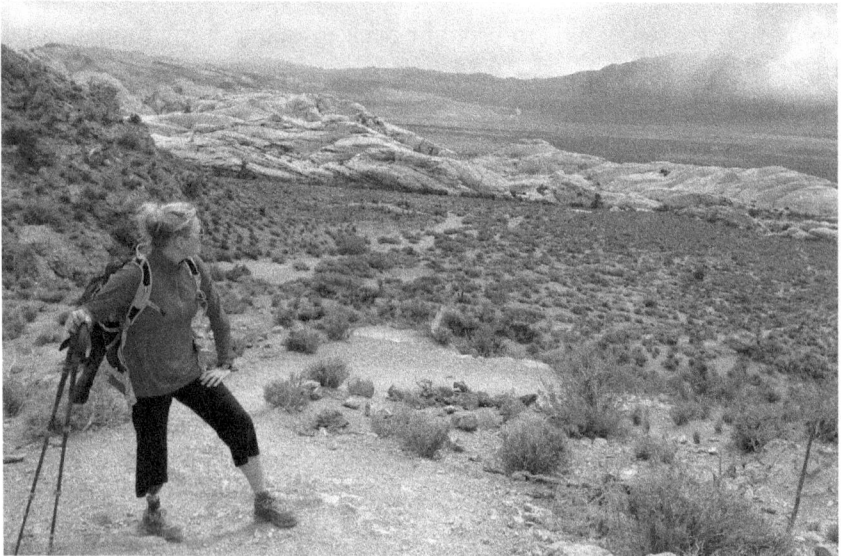

Contemplation of the storm in Red Rock Canyon, Las Vegas NV 2017.

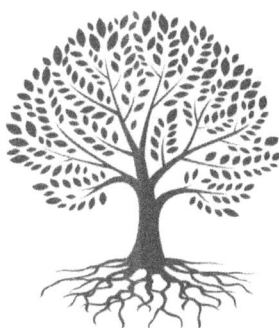

AFTERWORD

My situation and Chris's mirror each other in many ways: both professionals with a deep desire to help others, both mothers to two children, and both warriors of our unique health challenges. We both also possess a deep drive and determination to heal and be the best we can be—for ourselves, our children, and the world!

Either one of us could have easily thrown in the towel and given up when our health tumbled into crisis. But we made the choice to persevere each and every day, even when we thought we couldn't do it for even one more hour. We knew we didn't want to stay stagnant, and our children were watching our every move. So we pushed forward through the physical, mental, emotional, and spiritual storms because we want to inspire them to overcome, meet, and rise above the challenges, and help others on similar journeys.

I have faced my own battle with significant health challenges and chronic pain, intertwined with motherhood. In 2017, I was bed-ridden for many months due to a CSF leak. During that time, the pain, neurologic symptoms, and brain fog were at suffocating levels I hadn't experienced before. The mental gymnastics of my thoughts was debilitating in itself at times: "I have so much pain and fatigue, I can barely breathe. Yet, I know my children are relying on me, and I don't want to let them down. I want to be the strong, determined mother for them, but some days I just physically cannot do it!"

Thankfully, my husband, family, and friends helped carry the load as much as possible—they were such a gift and blessing during that time! I have spent the past six years healing and recovering. I'm not perfect now, but I'm doing so much better. Yet the thoughts of guilt and shame related to not being a good enough mother during those dark days and of how my illness has impacted my children's lives never go away.

Dealing with invisible illness and chronic pain as a mother and a healthcare provider is a unique situation. The patient in me is desperate for compassion, understanding, a solid plan of care, and relief! I've been frustrated at the lack of resources, the gaslighting, the "it's all in your head" and "learn to live with it" solutions. It feels like there should be a better way to help patients in these situations, besides just expecting us to deal with it.

The registered nurse in me feels like we are putting Band-Aids on the issues and shuffling people through the system like an assembly line. Some patients who need them are denied pain-relieving medications; others are given far too many and become addicted through no fault of their own. The system pushes medications for one issue that cause unwanted side effects, so a new medication is given to deal with the side effect of the first one. It's a vicious cycle! We desperately need to get to the root cause. We need to explore what support systems are in place; how overall health and wellness is related to sleep, nutrition, exercise, spirituality; and how these things impact chronic illness, pain, and quality of life.

As we continue to heal ourselves, it's important to help others who are stuck in the middle. We might not be able to heal the whole world, but by sharing our stories, we take the first steps toward helping others feel seen, heard, and valued. We are all a bit blessed and broken, trying to find our way into the light.

—Sara Bohling, MSN, RN
Nurse, coach, author of *When Grit and Grace Collide:*
Persevering Through Life's Challenges With Grit and God's Grace

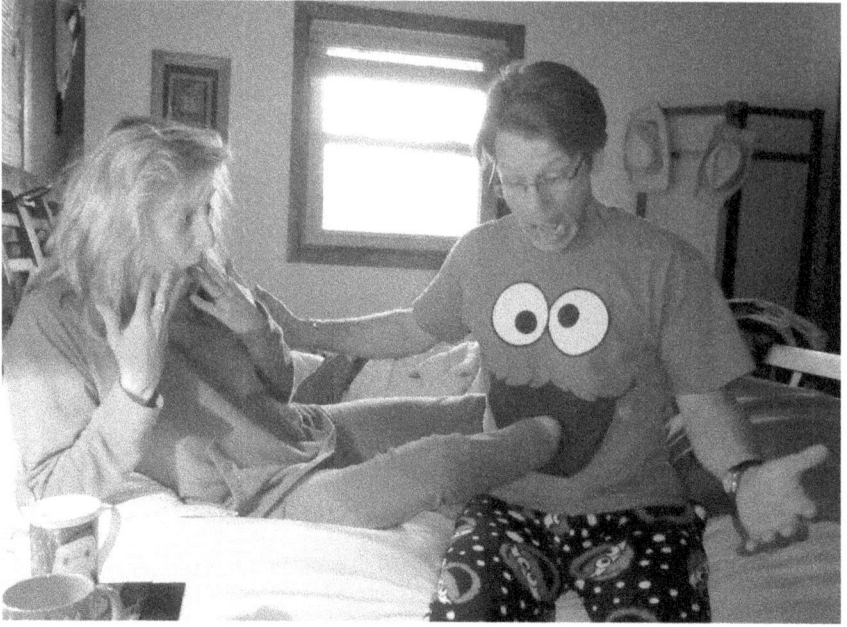

Oops, that's not a cookie! Nom nom nom (Chris and Scott circa 2017).

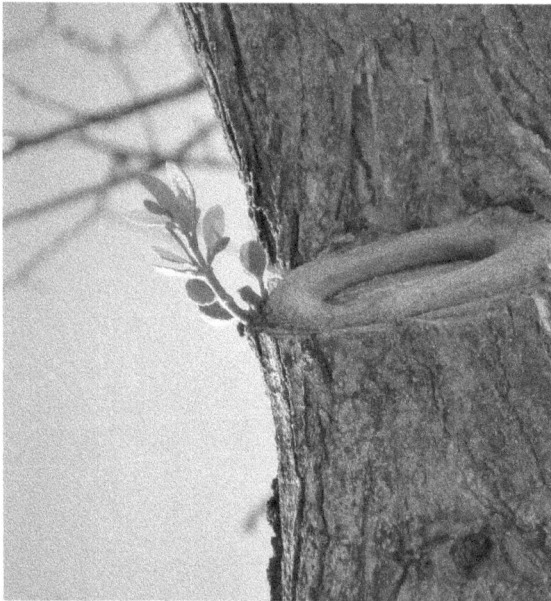

Sprouting new growth from loss, the Survivor Tree (Oklahoma City).

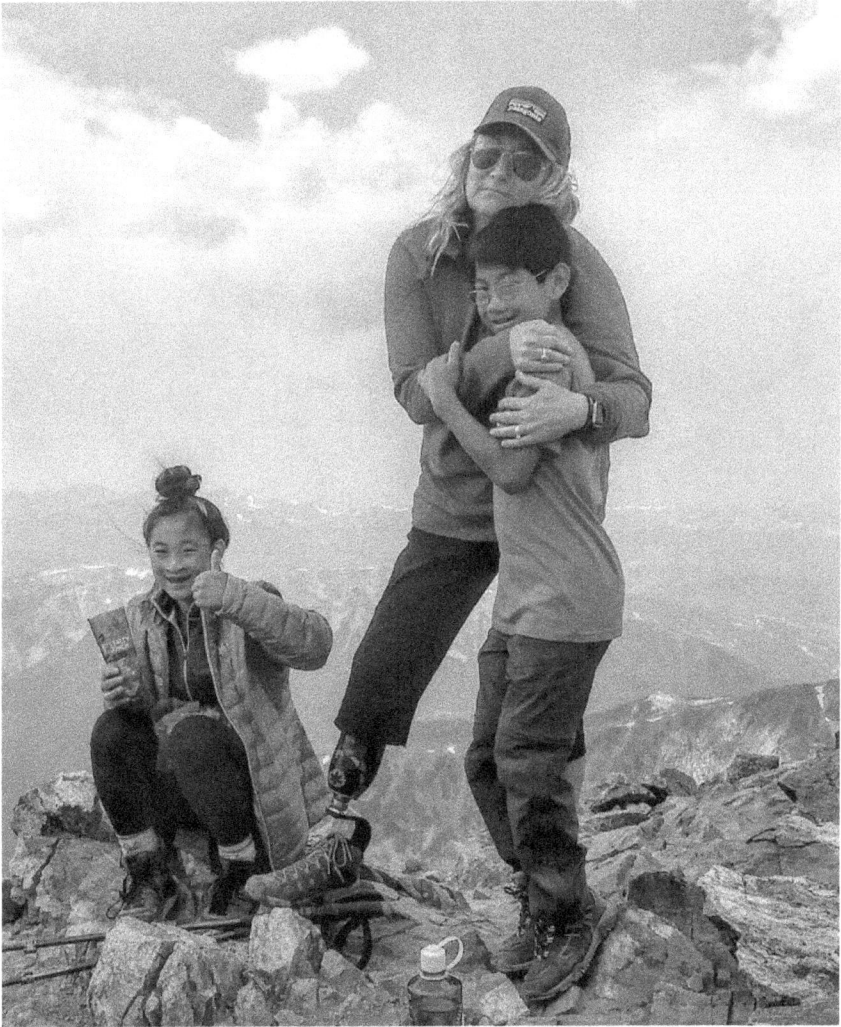

Gray's Peak (Colorado 14'er. Jade, Kai and Chris 2021).

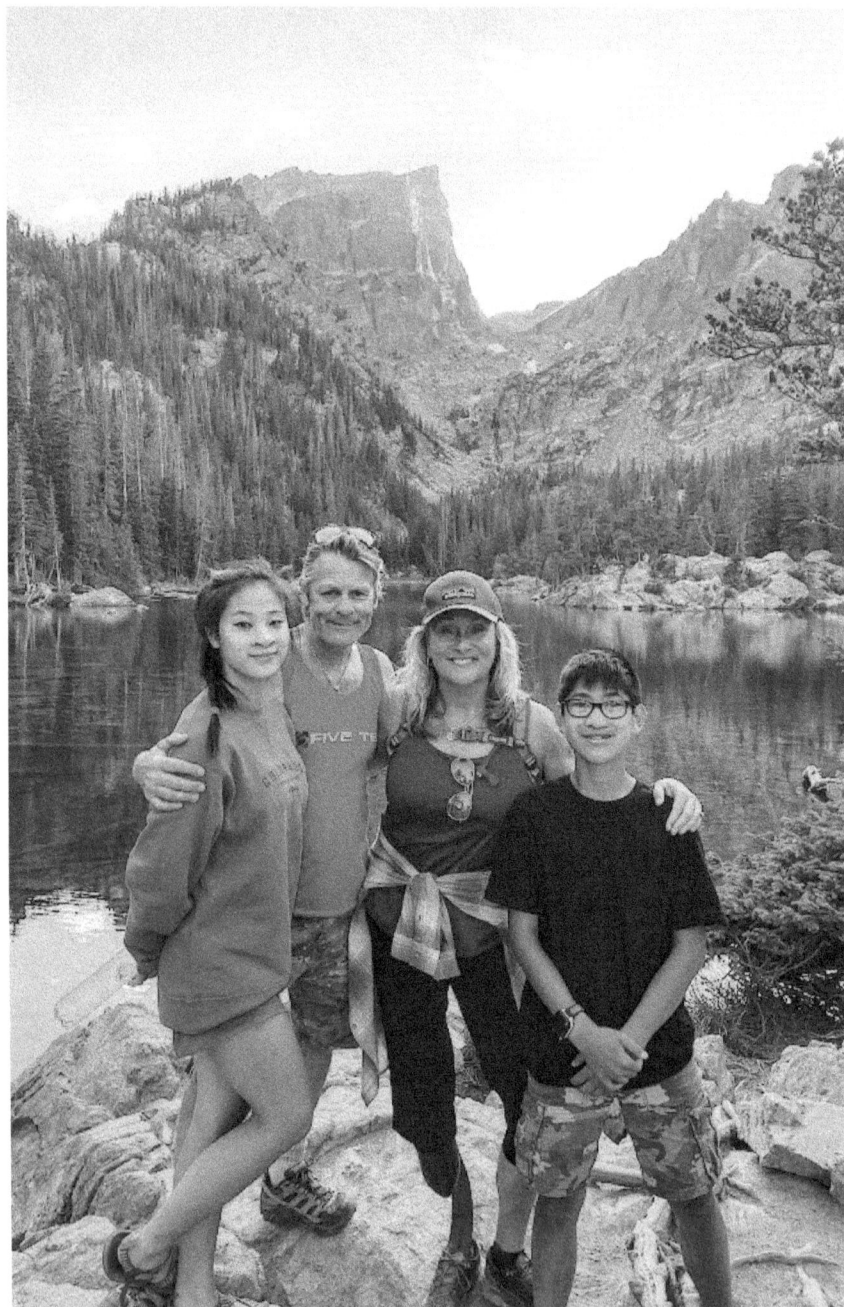

Jade, Scott, Chris and Kai at Rocky Mountain National Park, CO. 2022.

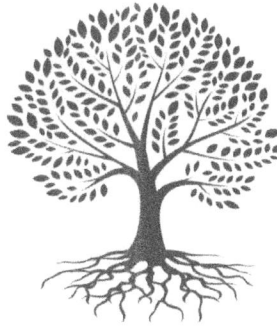

REFERENCES

American Heart Association. "How Does Depression Affect the Heart?" Last reviewed June 22, 2021. https://www.heart.org/en/healthy-living/healthy-lifestyle/mental-health-and-wellbeing/how-does-depression-affect-the-heart

American Psychological Association. "Exploring the mental health effects of poverty, hunger, and homelessness on children and teens." APA, last modified October 2022. https://www.apa.org/topics/socioeconomic-status/poverty-hunger-homelessness-children

Blewett, Kate, and Brian Woods. 1995. *The Dying Rooms*. Lauderdale Production. https://www.truevisiontv.com/films/the-dying-rooms-and-return

Child Welfare Information Gateway. 2017. "Supporting brain development in traumatized children and youth." Washington, D.C.: U.S. Department of Health and Human Services, Children's Bureau. https://www.childwelfare.gov/pubpdfs/braindevtrauma.pdf

Jauhar, Sandeep. 2018. *Heart: A History*. New York: Farrar, Straus and Giroux.

Nyaradi, Anett, Jianghong Li, Siobhan Hickling, Jonathan Foster, and Wendy H. Oddy. 2013 "The role of nutrition in children's neurocognitive development, from pregnancy through childhood." *Frontiers in Human Neuroscience* 7: Article 97. doi:10.3389/fnhum.2013.00097

Prange-Morgan, Chris. 2018. "What Nobody Tells You About Parenting a Child With a History of Extreme Trauma." *Huffington Post.* https://www.huffpost.com/entry/parenting-a-child-with-a-history-of-extreme-trauma_n_5acf7a3de4b0edca2cb7357b

Rankin, Arthur, and Jules Bass. 1970. *Santa Claus Is Coming to Town.* Rankin and Bass Productions.

Schroeder, Lisa. 2019. "Pittsburgh Foundation issues public comment against changes to SNAP." *The Pittsburgh Foundation*, September 9. https://pittsburghfoundation.org/snap-comments-2019#:~:text=Hunger%2Drelated%20toxic%20stress%20can,less%20during%20the%20school%20year

Shah, Anuj. K., Sendhil Mullainathan, and Eldar Shafir. 2012. "Some consequences of having too little." *Science*, 338:682–685. doi:10.1126/science.1222426

Silverstein, Shel. 1964. *The Giving Tree.* New York: Harper Collins.

Simmons, Philip. 2002. *Learning to Fall: The Blessings of an Imperfect Life.* New York: Bantam.

Spicuzza, Mary. 2019. "Milwaukee is the most racially segregated metro area in the country, Brookings report says." *Milwaukee Journal Sentinel*, January 8. https://www.jsonline.com/story/news/local/milwaukee/2019/01/08/milwaukee-most-segregated-area-country-brookings-says/2512258002/

The TODAY Show. 2018. "How Mommy Burnout Led This 'Trauma Mama' to a Serious Injury." NBC. https://www.today.com/video/

how-mommy-burnout-led-this-trauma-mama-to-a-serious-injury-1218786883962

Thiel, Kali. 2015. "Sheboygan Native Helps Disabled After Climbing Injury." *Sheboygan Press*, July 17. https://www.sheboyganpress.com/story/news/local/2015/07/17/climbing-amputee/30323733/

Van der Kolk, Bessel. 2015. *The Body Keeps the Score: Brain, Mind and Body in the Healing of Trauma*. New York: Penguin Publishing Group.

Verrier, Nancy. 1993. *The Primal Wound: Understanding the Adopted Child*. Baltimore: Gateway Press.

Winfrey, Oprah and Bruce Perry. 2021. *What Happened to You? Conversations on Trauma, Resilience, and Healing*. Flatiron Books. https://static.macmillan.com/static/fib/what-happened-to-you/

Winnicott, Donald. 1975. "Transitional Objects and Transitional Phenomena (1951)." *Through Paediatrics to Psychoanalysis: Collected Papers*, 229–242. https://psptraining.com/wp-content/uploads/Winnicott-D.W.-1958.-Through-paediatrics-to-psycho-analysis.pdf

Wise, Roy A. and Mykel A. Robble. 2020. "Dopamine and Addiction." *Annual Review of Psychology*, 71:79–106. doi:10.1146/annurev-psych-010418-103337

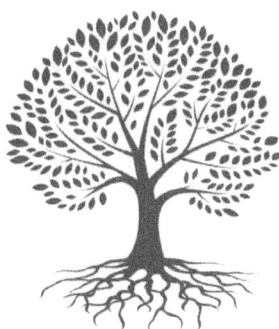

RESOURCES

Adaptive Adventures. https://adaptiveadventures.org/

Adaptively Abled. https://www.adaptivelyabledamputees.org/

The Amp'd Up 211 Podcast (featuring individuals in the limb loss community). https://ampup211.com/

Amplitude Magazine (for those living with limb loss). https://livingwithamplitude.com/

Amputee Coalition. https://www.amputee-coalition.org/

Association for Clinical Pastoral Education. https://acpe.edu/

Care for Children International, Inc. https://drfederici.com/

Carrie O'Toole Ministries. https://carrieotoole.com/

Catalyst Sports. https://catalystsports.org/

Center for Disease Control and Prevention (CDC) *What is Early Intervention?* (last reviewed August 9th, 2022) What is "Early Intervention"? | CDC

Challenged Athletes Foundation. https://www.challengedathletes.org.

CPTSD Foundation: The Foundation for Post-Traumatic Healing and Complex Trauma Research. https://cptsdfoundation.org/

Early Intervention, CDC. https://www.cdc.gov/ncbddd/actearly/parents/states.html

Great Lakes Adaptive Sports Association (GLASA). https://www.glasa.org/

Lifespan Trauma Consulting. https://lifespantrauma.com/

Love Without Boundaries. https://www.lovewithoutboundaries.com/

No Barriers. https://nobarriersusa.org/

Paradox Sports. https://www.paradoxsports.org/

Profound Awesomeness: A Podcast by Adrian Jones. https://profoundawesomeness.com/

RAD Sibs (for siblings impacted by Reactive Attachment Disorder). https://radsibs.org/

RAD Advocates (for caregivers/professionals working with children with Reactive Attachment Disorder). https://www.radadvocates.org/

RAD Talk with Tracey. https://www.radtalkwithtracey.com/

Team River Runner. https://www.teamriverrunner.org/

The Underground World of RAD Facebook Page. https://www.facebook.com/groups/344527186042906

Wisconsin Department of Health Services Birth to Three Program. https://dhs.wisconsin.gov/birthto3/index.htm

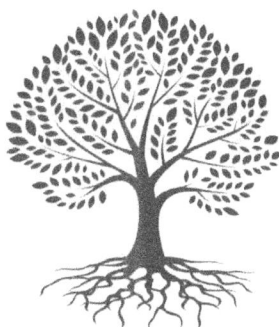

FURTHER READING

Bartasius, Elizabeth. 2019. *The Elegant Out: A Novel*. She Writes Press.

Bohling, Sara. 2022. *When Grit and Grace Collide: Persevering Through Life's Challenges With Grit and God's Grace*. Independently Published.

Bowler, Kate. 2018. *Everything Happens for a Reason and Other Lies I've Loved*. Random House. https://katebowler.com/books/everything-happens-for-a-reason/

Cain, Susan. 2022. *Bittersweet: How Sorrow and Longing Make Us Whole*. Crown. https://susancain.net/book/bittersweet/

Grace, Jenn. 2020. *House on Fire: Finding Resilience, Hope and Purpose in the Ashes*. Publish Your Purpose Press. https://jenntgrace.com/house-on-fire-finding-resilience-hope-and-purpose-in-the-ashes/

Knipper, Stephanie. 2017. *The Peculiar Miracles of Antoinette Martin*. Workman Publishing. https://www.workman.com/products/the-peculiar-miracles-of-antoinette-martin/paperback

McCormick, Tim. 2015. "Still Hanging On." *Milwaukee Magazine*, March 11. https://www.milwaukeemag.com/still-hanging-on-ada ptive-adventures/

Nelson, Joanne. 2020. *This is How We Leave*. Vine Leaves Press. https://www.vineleavespress.com/this-is-how-we-leave-by-joanne-nelson.html.

Oberholtzer, Janet. 2015. *Because I Can: Doing What I Can, With What I Have, Where I Am*. Createspace. https://www.amazon.com/Because-Can-Doing-What-Where/dp/1514283921

Prange-Morgan, Chris. 2018. "What Nobody Tells You About Parenting a Child With a History of Extreme Trauma." *Huffington Post*. https://www.huffpost.com/entry/parenting-a-child-with-a-history-of-extreme-trauma_n_5acf7a3de4b0edca2cb7357b

Prange-Morgan, Chris. 2022. "Why 'Good Enough' Parenting Is Better Than Perfection." *Psychology Today*. https://www.psychologytoday.com/us/blog/full-catastrophe-parenting/202208/why-good-enough-parenting-is-better-perfection

Seung Chan Lim. 2013. *Realizing Empathy: An Inquiry Into the Meaning of Making*. https://realizingempathy.com/books/

Thiel, Kali. 2015. "Sheboygan Native Helps Disabled After Climbing Injury." *Sheboygan Press*, July 17. https://www.sheboyganpress.com/story/news/local/2015/07/17/climbing-amputee/30323733/

Williams, Keri. 2022. *but, he spit in my coffee: A reads-like-fiction memoir about adopting a child with Reactive Attachment Disorder (RAD)*. Independently Published. https://keri-williams.com/

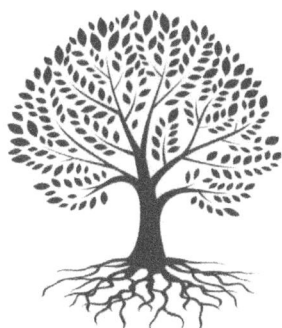

CONNECT WITH CHRIS

To learn more about Chris Prange-Morgan, visit
ChrisPrangeMorgan.com

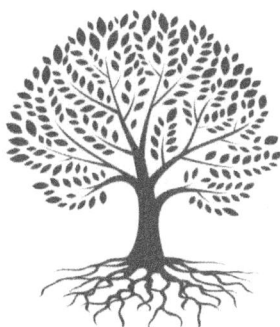

ABOUT THE AUTHOR

Chris Prange-Morgan, MA, MSW, considers herself a student of all types of trauma. Before becoming a parent to her children, Prange-Morgan worked for more than ten years as a mental health professional and social worker with adults in the criminal justice system. She has a master's degree in social work from Loyola University Chicago, a certificate of advanced graduate study in pastoral counseling from Neuman College, and a master of arts in religious studies from Cardinal Stritch University. Prange-Morgan has sought to better understand collective and generational trauma and its effect on individuals after she suffered a life-changing accident in 2011, becoming a trauma survivor herself. Her story has been featured on *The Today Show*, *The Trauma Therapist Project*, CBS, *Milwaukee Magazine*, *The Institute for Healthcare Improvement* website, *The No Barriers Podcast*, and *The Conversation Project*. Her articles have appeared in many publications, including *Psychology Today*, *Huffington Post*, *Able Outdoors*, and *Living With Amplitude Magazine*. She and her husband have coached parents and professionals in the trenches of working with challenging life and family circumstances.

The B Corp Movement

Dear reader,

Thank you for reading this book and joining the Publish Your Purpose community! You are joining a special group of people who aim to make the world a better place.

What's Publish Your Purpose About?

Our mission is to elevate the voices often excluded from traditional publishing. We intentionally seek out authors and storytellers with diverse backgrounds, life experiences, and unique perspectives to publish books that will make an impact in the world.

Certified

(B)

®

Corporation

Beyond our books, we are focused on tangible, action-based change. As a woman- and LGBTQ+-owned company, we are committed to reducing inequality, lowering levels of poverty, creating a healthier environment, building stronger communities, and creating high-quality jobs with dignity and purpose.

As a Certified B Corporation, we use business as a force for good. We join a community of mission-driven companies building a more equitable, inclusive, and sustainable global economy. B Corporations must meet high standards of transparency, social and environmental performance, and accountability as determined by the nonprofit B Lab. The certification process is rigorous and ongoing (with a recertification requirement every three years).

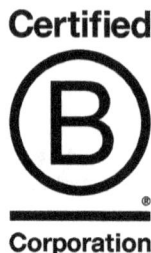

How Do We Do This?

We intentionally partner with socially and economically disadvantaged businesses that meet our sustainability goals. We embrace and encourage our authors and employee's differences in race, age, color, disability, ethnicity, family or marital status, gender identity or expression, language, national origin, physical and mental ability, political affiliation, religion, sexual orientation, socio-economic status, veteran status, and other characteristics that make them unique.

Community is at the heart of everything we do—from our writing and publishing programs to contributing to social enterprise nonprofits like reSET (https://www.resetco.org/) and our work in founding B Local Connecticut.

We are endlessly grateful to our authors, readers, and local community for being the driving force behind the equitable and sustainable world we are building together.

To connect with us online, or publish with us,
visit us at www.publishyourpurpose.com.

Elevating Your Voice,

Jenn T. Grace

Jenn T. Grace
Founder, Publish Your Purpose

www.ingramcontent.com/pod-product-compliance
Lightning Source LLC
Chambersburg PA
CBHW020608270326
41927CB00005B/233